# Become a
# Medical Intuitive

*The Complete Developmental Course*

## SECOND EDITION

## Tina M. Zion

Virginia

Published by WriteLife Publishing
(an Imprint of Boutique of Quality Books Publishing Company)
www.writelife.com

Printed in the United States of America

978-1-60808-199-8 (p)
978-1-60808-200-1 (e)

Library of Congress Control Number: 2018951087

Book design by Robin Krauss, www.bookformatters.com
Cover artwork by Corey Ford, www.coreyfordgallery.com

Editor: Olivia Swenson

# Contents

## Part One

## Part Two

# Part Three

# PART ONE

## You and the Universe

# Chapter 1

## Medical Intuitition Welcomes You

My closed eyes popped open in shock. I had just perceived a woman's lungs as if I were an x-ray machine! I saw the individual tissue and the alveoli (tiny air sacks within the lungs) in their grape-like clusters. Inflamed orange-red energy filled her lungs, the right side much more irritated than the left. I could see darkened areas within the red. It had taken a few minutes of observation before I realized I was peering inside this woman's body, deep into her lungs.

"Are you a smoker?"

"Oh yeah, I plan to quit soon," she declared with a laugh.

We were surrounded by thirty or so other women, all taking a break during a weekend workshop. I was one of the presenters for the program, but as I look back, I am no longer sure what the program was even about. At that moment I became a medical intuitive. The retreat center and all the lively, talkative women around me just faded away.

That experience of looking into another human's lungs like a photographer taking a digital image or an x-ray machine showing a troubled area—that was the beginning. The medical realm of intuition continued to increase after that. With each session following that moment, I saw tissue, organs, cancer, psychic surgery, tumors, broken bones, deceased relatives, guardian angels, and spirit guides, and I received messages from beyond. The more energy work I did, the stronger and clearer the information came in.

I was so intrigued with my perceptions that I began to insist on checking in with my client's energy field before they told me anything regarding their physical body or their emotional state. Beyond initial hellos, I would not let them describe anything about themselves. I thought this was the only way that people would believe me and the level of accuracy I was achieving. Looking back, I think I was the only one questioning it!

In 1979, I sat down for lunch with a physician's wife in the hospital where we both worked. She was obviously in distress, complaining that her sinuses were so congested she could not breathe. She went on to say that the pressure came on suddenly, out of nowhere. I instantly blurted out, "That is tears you are stuffing down, and you need to let yourself cry." The astounded look on her face told me I had spoken a deep truth to this woman and she was not prepared for it, especially in such a public setting. While I knew I was correct, I felt that I could have taken a more sensitive approach. Even then, prior to any mind-body training, I instinctively knew the cause of her illness.

The more accurate I became as a medical intuitive, the more driven I was to write a book about it. I examined my intuitive processes and the processes that took place for my clients. I examined each session from the first moment of contact with my clients until the last moment as they walked out of my office. Over and over again, for many months, I took note of each tiny detail as it happened.

I questioned myself throughout the process. *What am I feeling? What is going on now? How does it feel when I experience another's energy field so intimately? What happens within my own body? How am I receiving the pure essence of this person's medical issue? Through what sense does the information come through? Do I see it, feel it, hear it, smell it, or does the information come in waves of knowing or waves of instant thought?* I logged the insights that evolved during those sessions with my clients. That log became the foundation for this book and the outline for my weekend workshop.

You do not need a medical background to do medical intuition. This book will take you through progressive, step-by-step training as a medical intuitive. Like my weekend workshop, "Become a Medical Intuitive: The Complete Developmental Course," this book is jam-packed with guided experiences, actual case studies, and new ways to understand your natural abilities. Each page provides you with an enriched learning experience.

You too can learn to be a medical intuitive. Read the cases, study the tables and diagrams, and put the experiences into practice. If it seems right for you to read the book through first and then go back to the beginning to take action with each step, do it. Or you might prefer to do each practice assignment as you first read through the book. Notice already that I am asking you to assess your own instincts and follow your own guidance. This is crucial for your development. I am only the guide along your journey as an emerging medical intuitive.

I have personally experienced heightened success when I work with a study partner. Having a partner keeps each of you on track and keeps you accountable. You can work with a partner over the phone as I did for more than two years, or you might find someone locally who is interested in excelling as a medical intuitive. You can both agree to read certain pages and work through the awareness assignments. As you progress further into the course, you can then work with each other's energy.

Take the time to document your development throughout this process. You will not be able to consciously remember it all. Purchase a notebook specifically for your medical intuition evolvement. Many times throughout this book I ask you to describe or to draw your perceptions. Your most accurate information will come in flashes, so you must document everything along the way. Log those perceptions in writing so you will remember each step of your expanding awareness.

As you write in your journal, also write in this book. Really make it yours. Learn and write. Write and learn. Use this book and take action with what you learn. Like my workshop, this book is set up as a progressive, step-by-step course to promote confidence without performance anxiety.

Our Western state-of-the-art medical system does not delve into the cause of illness or the creation of disease. Our medical system is astounding at finding and diagnosing disease, but methods of discovering how the disease developed or what factors helped create the illness seem nonexistent. While allopathic medicine understands that stress may cause a stomach ulcer, it does not take it to the next steps. If the mind-body connection can make us sick, it can also make us well.

My focus for this book centers on accessing detailed mind-body information for the benefit of the individual who is receiving the information. Medical intuition accesses mental, emotional, and physical interconnections and retrieves the hidden aspects of ailments or disease that allopathic medicine cannot discern with laboratory tests and procedures. Medical intuition looks at the symptoms but ventures beyond, going to the source of an illness.

## The Medical Intuitive Within You

Humans are glowing balls of electromagnetic abilities, understanding, and insights. We have the ability to heal ourselves and to assist others in their healing. Trust, understand, and honor your innate intuitive strengths and the ability to put them to work for our personal well-being and the well-being of all. Begin right now. Be fascinated with anything that you become aware of. There is no right or wrong as you grow in your own unique awareness.

Medical intuitives discover hidden and unconscious truths within multidimensional patterns, vibrating in complex relationships with the human body. Medical intuition is one of the most therapeutic of all the healing modalities. When you help an ill person understand the essence beneath their issues and struggles, you will see a face brighten or you will hear the "aha" in their voice. Time and time again you will see a sparkle in the eyes of an ill person that only moments ago were clouded with worry or fear. As you share your intuitive knowledge, you will see your awareness provide meaningful insights, which give relief and healing. People simply want to understand what is happening to them, why it is happening, and what they can do about it.

Medical intuition is an art that can be learned and then polished into precision. I became an accurate medical intuitive because,

I tuned into people every single day. In other words, practice, practice, practice, notice, notice, notice. More practice brings forth more accuracy. Don't just think about intuition as you read this book . . . participate and take action with it.

## Medical Intuition as a Healing Technique

I want to emphasize that profound healing does take place during medical intuitive sessions. People who come to intuitives are often so tired and so perplexed about their malady or their disease. They are often desperate for help and as a result are open to intuitive information that under normal circumstances they would never be open to. By the time they come to you, they have often exhausted all other possibilities. People, in general, need to talk about their struggles and are fascinated when they receive intuitive information about their issues.

Tony stepped into my office for a reading. He appeared to be in his late twenties, healthy, trim, and muscular. As we settled into the chairs and I received permission from him to enter into his story, I quickly noticed his chest felt tight, constricted, and full of anxiety. As I described the tightness, he nodded his head in agreement. Here is a portion of the transcript of our conversation:

**Tina:** I am picking up some anxiety, some anxiousness, some clenching down. I am picking up two balls of energy that are coming together and intermingling. This could be two issues or two people, you in a relationship. The balls of energy looked like they would come together and then blow up, but they didn't. They came together, interlacing with each other. You are touching in with emotions that you have not been connecting with. I literally saw your finger reaching out and touching water; water is a symbol for emotion. You are touching in with your emotions and just watching the ripples.

Again, I am concerned about tightness and anxiety—touching in with this emotion, something new. I see the symbol of a flower with an empty center. The center is not in full growth and somehow it is hollow and empty. I see that you are nodding with the comment I just made. The touching in with emotion and the full bloom of the flower makes it look to others like you are rocking and rolling but on the inside you are empty.

**Tony:** Yes.

**Tina:** On the outside you look to other people like you've got it going and you are in charge, but on the inside you feel like something is missing.

**Tony:** Yes, a deeper desire.

**Tina:** Yes, something missing. I just got goose bumps and that always tells me that I just mentioned a deep truth and you connected with this truth. Does this make any sense to you?

**Tony:** Yes.

**Tina:** I am concerned about this flower . . . the full bloom of the flower. I can go down inside of the flower's center and I should not be able to. It looks like an empty tunnel.

**Tony:** Yes, a flower came up in a reading from someone else. They saw a flower coming up out of concrete. I was finding my spiritual self even through difficulties. Lately I have been pushing for deeper understanding because I am not where I want to be. I know there is something still there to figure out. I have been pushing and it has been painful. It takes everything I thought I knew and now I have to look at it again. When I accept a new reality it takes the magic out of it . . . a little bit of the fantasy that in 3D everyone enjoys. It takes a little bit of that away so now I am relearning.

**Tina:** I see a superhuman cape on your shoulders, but then you show me the empty flower and I have to keep mentioning the emptiness. It depends on what you consider magic. In the Bible miracles were happening all over the place and people nowadays want to know what happened to all the miracles. When something looks like a miracle it is really just following the laws of the universe. A lot of times people are disappointed and say, "Where did the magic go?" The more you learn, the more you realize that you need to learn. But also the more you learn, you realize that some of the universe is almost mechanical and it takes the magic out of it. We learn how things work together or don't work together . . . how things fit or don't fit.

**Tony:** Yes.

**Tina:** Tell me about this clenching and anxiety in your heart and gut.

**Tony:** I have been working on getting closer to the source, to get the true understanding for as long as I can stay in this body. My hope and desire is to truly understand that and to show other people. But now I am questioning more and trying to figure out where I fit in.

**Tina:** As I look at your energy field at this moment, your head is a glowball. You are quite a thinker, and also the right and left hemispheres of your brain are very equal. You can analyze the details on the left hemisphere and on the right you can grasp the magic, grasp the bigger concepts. I am telling you, your head is fired up and very bright and you have a lot of confidence and vitality because I see a great deal of orange.

As I check out the rest of you there is no glow around your heart. When I saw your finger touch the surface of the water, you are beginning to make the connections about all of this awareness, but your heart is not as advanced in its development as your thinking is. It is not linking together like it could be. It is overshadowed. You are holding back and clenching down in the heart area. It is not shining out like both sides of your head are. Does this make sense to you?

**Tony:** That is the missing piece! I am not feeling it!

**Tina:** No, you are not feeling it.

**Tony:** No.

**Tina:** Let me check this more. You are even expressing well because your throat is as alive and bright as your head, but the cut off is right here. (Tina motions to the chest area between the throat and the heart.)

**Tony:** That is the missing piece. It makes sense because I have been working on my head and throat area to open up. I couldn't feel the pain and scarring. The missing piece is going from conceptualized thinking and knowing and getting to believing. In order to get there, I have to experience it and feel it.

**Tina:** You have to feel it.

**Tony:** Yeah and I have to feel it before I can believe. I can read and think and get so far. I am trying to figure out how to get here, I guess. (He points to his heart chakra.)

**Tina:** Really knowing something is not all about the books. It's that full-bodied, full-mind sense. You have relied deeply on your head, but this is about the knowing of it. Let me check this out for you . . . Your finger is only touching the very surface of the water . . . the surface of feeling. What is keeping you on the surface? You are busy watching the ripples along the surface but you are not willing to dive in.

**Tony:** It is fear I am sure.

**Tina:** That takes us back to the clenching down in your heart center.

**Tony:** In my meditations I would get right to my heart but then I thought that I would die . . . that my physical heart would stop. It would go crazy so then I would stop the meditation because I thought I was leaving (dying). That means unfinished business for me. I think Spirit was meeting me halfway and now I am having a hard time getting back.

**Tina:** I am seeing an eye that is three-fourths closed. Your heart center is only a fourth of the way open. I will ask what your heart needs. (Short pause.) I am hearing, "It really is okay to feel the fire. It is okay to let it be fired up." They say they want you to practice allowing your heart to be fired up. You can do this as you drive down the road or in the shower. Do it right now. Feel it fire up like a car's engine. Fired up and turning over. Do it right now.

**Tony:** This is strangely difficult.

**Tina:** Try again, but don't try so hard and I will watch as you do it. See a nice campfire, under control . . . not sparking all over the place but under control and ready for hotdogs and marshmallows. I see a trickle of it beginning now, but you are trying to start a fire that is sitting on a swamp of old muck, old emotion instead of dry, solid ground. You have old emotions that are keeping your fire too damp.

**Tony:** It's been hard to move on and turn the page. It's about the mother of my child . . .

Tony and I continued a gentle process of stirring around in the emotional muck. Working together, he noticed, felt, and explored his emotions in a non-threatening way. He didn't have to push his emotions down as he had been doing and he didn't have to do it alone. I was there with a safety net of calm, asking him to experience his feelings. By the time he left, he was able to move around in his constricted heart energy. The spark of life reignited and his heart energy increased and expanded once again. I described to him how his heart energy became brighter and clearer as he participated in this medical intuitive session. I could see his energy change as we stirred around in his old pain. I described the new glow to him as it changed during this process.

Medical intuition is a healing process. As you offer intuitive information, you can also psychically watch the individual's energy change. As the person listens and incorporates the intuitive information you share, you will be able to see and experience their energy shifting. You can share the energy changes with the individual as it happens. This is the power of medical intuition.

This book and medical intuition is not about fighting against Western medicine. It is about cooperative systems working together for the well-being of the individual. It is integrative medicine at its finest.

## A Brief History of Medical Intuition

Medical intuition has been around since people have been around. Shamans, medicine men, midwives, and herbalists have existed since humans have been on Earth. These prominent leaders throughout time are the original medical intuitives. The wisdom and the traditions were never placed into print. Like this book and the course, the ancient healers taught apprentices through hands-on experience and the discussion of each experience.

It was not until the 1840s that John Elliotson, MD, (1791–1868) author of *Surgical Operations in the Mesmeric State without Pain* (1843), actually documented using a trance state to medically diagnose another human being. Most people interested in alternative health have already heard of Edgar Cayce. In the late 1800s Edgar Cayce became a phenomenally famous medical diagnostician using only the information that came to him through a deep altered state.

In 2000, I heard a presentation by Dr. Norm Shealy, a Harvard-trained neurosurgeon, at the US Psychotronics Association Conference in Louisville, Kentucky, in which Dr. Shealy stated he had coined the term "medical intuitive." Now a myriad of others publicly recognize the mind-body connection. Herbert Benson, a Harvard researcher, is well known for his discoveries regarding meditation. His findings show meditation's positive effect on stress in the physical body. Candace Pert, scientist and author of *Molecules of Emotion*, has found evidence of a mind-body connection possibly created by a release and absorption of neuro-peptides. In other words, what we think creates a chemical response within our body and brain. In some of her writings she refers to this connection between body and mind with the term "body-mind."

In her book *Everything You Need to Know to Feel Go(o)d*, Pert states: "We can't deny that the body and mind are one, tied by cellular receptors strewn throughout the matrix and vibrating to create waves of emotion and information. The body doesn't exist only to carry the head around."

## Five Ethical Issues

Suddenly I was traveling through a tunnel of pinkish membrane. I thought, *What the heck is this and what am I doing?* My guide was sending me on an intestinal journey! This was a surprise I have not forgotten. As I zoomed through my client's intestines. I began to see some lumps and bumpiness that did not look like the rest of the intestinal wall. The bumps were nearly black in color. They stuck up from the wall like short, stubby fingers. My inner vision saw the stubby fingers within the colon, on the right side of her lower abdomen. The energy field of my own body felt a huge, bulging thickness in her energy field at that same location.

I did not say, "Mary, you are at the beginning stages of colon cancer." I did describe to her what I saw and felt and asked her to promise me she would call her doctor that day and ask for a colonoscopy. Mary followed through immediately. Not only that, but she took my drawing of her energy field to her doctor's appointment and showed it to him. Thank goodness he did not dismiss this seventy-eight-year-old woman and her "quack" energy worker. He followed through with the colonoscopy and found a large group of polyps just beginning to turn cancerous. They were removed and Mary recovered quickly.

### Essential Point:
*Never give a medical diagnosis if you are not an MD.*

My experience with Mary is a great example of allopathic medicine and non-traditional, holistic medicine working together in harmony and for the good of each individual.

We will now look at five ethical issues, listed below, in more detail, including my own opinion of how each issue should be resolved. Each of these points are important to remember as you begin your own work.

1. Giving a medical diagnosis

2. Discouraging people from traditional medicine

3. Asking permission in medical intuition

4. Telling people about intuitive information received

5. Receiving money or barter for the spiritual work you do

**Giving a medical diagnosis.** Never give a medical diagnosis to your client under any circumstances. Only physicians are licensed to diagnosis. You can, however, thoroughly describe what you see and feel. Describe your perceptions in precise detail but without labels or anything that might be considered a medical diagnosis.

Do not get bogged down in trying to interpret your intuitive insights. In fact, do not offer any interpretations. Ask the client what your insights mean to them. You will be constantly surprised when people tell you that they know exactly what you sense and what it means to them. Simply describe the information that comes to you.

Describe, describe, and describe in exact precise detail. Notice how describing is different from a diagnostic label.

**Discouraging people from traditional medicine.** Never discourage people from traditional medicine. I often find myself asking my client to call their physician right after our session and request an appointment or a specific medical test to determine what I have just perceived intuitively. True integrative medicine incorporates many holistic and spiritual modalities with Western medicine.

**Asking permission in medical intuition.** We must get permission first! Without permission, the psychic or medical intuitive is breaking and entering into our "body-home." Our body and energy field is our sacred space that no one should enter physically or intuitively without permission. I do not intuitively push myself on anyone who does not approach me with the request. Sometimes asking someone verbally for permission is not an option, but it is always an option to ask for permission on an intuitive level. I frequently ask people telepathically for their permission. You must honor their wishes when you receive a no from someone.

My new grandbaby is an example. He has been fraught with physical struggles since his birth. Regardless of his newborn age, I asked him for permission to energetically assist him. Yes, even a newborn has the right to say yes or no, and we must abide by those responses. No, I did not ask his parents for permission. Each of us is an individual, even as we are born into this earthly world. This little baby is his own being, and I must honor his wishes. He did say yes, but if I had received a no I would have had to honor that as well.

When I received his permission, I instantly received a vision of him in the tiny hospital crib. In my mind's eye, I stepped closer to him, but I instantly jumped back again. He was rising up as if levitating on a magic carpet. When I looked more closely I realized the magic carpet was really a small blanket that stretched out forming a type of trampoline. Three young male angels were stretching this energetic blanket between them and our struggling little baby was being tossed up and down in the air. Each time he was catapulted upward, they skillfully caught him again in the blanket. The three teenager angels continued to toss him upward and catch him in the blanket on the way down.

While it seemed that the angels were aware of my presence, they continued to propel him over and over in a rhythmic pattern similar to his rhythm of breathing. My grandbaby was laughing loudly and throwing his tiny arms and legs while airborne. He then looked quite pleased each time he landed back in the blanket. To this day I have no idea how this related to my attempting a medical intuitive scan. Even though his death seemed imminent, I began to chuckle with the four of them and their antics. Our baby did not pass on and in fact is doing well at the time of this writing.

**Essential Point:**
*Our body and energy field is our sacred space.*

Receiving a no from someone does not mean you will always receive a no. Wait a day or two or even a week and check again.

I have received a "No, do not enter!" for days in a row only to later receive a jovial "*Yes!*" from that same person. Our souls dwell in a profoundly involved experience and we have no idea of their complexity. Who are we to interfere and push forward for someone when all signals say to stand back?

Time and time again I hear justifications from clients and fans on my Facebook pages to push on without permission. The fans declare that we must help the individual anyway because it can do no harm. Well, have you noticed that people are amazing at justifying just about anything they do? Breaking and entering into a home usually does not end up physically harming the homeowners, but they are still violated.

Even when you have a powerful urge to push into someone else's experience to "help them out," stop yourself. Do not try to justify the healing or the energy that you desperately wish to give your family, friend, or neighbor. Honoring all the refusals that you receive verbally or intuitively will prevent you from shifting into the negative or darker side of energy work. People who work from the darker side of energy work do not request permission.

I declare again and again, "Ask for permission." When we ask for permission, all kinds of things begin to happen. The energy of caring touches another's energy field in some unconscious way. That person does make an unconscious decision to receive or not receive the assistance. But there is more. The request for permission establishes a signal of respect for the individual. That signal of respect has substance and is recognized on an energetic level, and thus a soul level.

When that person sends a "Yes, come right on in," something else takes place. That person begins to actively participate with the experience of receiving. Actively participating, consciously or unconsciously, opens a wider energetic door to healing, which in turn improves and even accelerates the receiver's own process.

Try this approach. Intuitively ask, from your soul's heart to the heart of the potential receiver, for permission to assist them. Do not rely on your mind because our minds are controlling and can rationalize and defend just about anything.

When you are able to intuitively ask for consent from the very soul essence of another, you have turned it over to the receiving person and have made it less about you and more about them. So yes, I agree that we can do no harm sending love and healing to someone in need and if they do not want it, it will probably just bounce away to someone who does. Requesting permission first, however, no matter what the situation is, brings honor and grace to both the receiver and the healer.

**Telling people about intuitive information received.** I do have a rule about this. Only inform your client if they agree to hear your intuitive information. Do not surprise a person by giving them intuitive information that they did not ask for. Do not go up to them in a shopping mall or the grocery. If you approach them unexpectedly they will be surprised or even shocked. They may not be ready to hear what you received. Do not make this about you being an intuitive. Make this about the other person. Be sensitive for them. If you want to approach someone, the key is to open the door by simply asking the person what they think of the spirit world or what they feel about it. Their response will tell you if you can proceed in sharing your intuitive insight with them. If the person is a client, please tell them that you received some intuitive information and ask if they would like to hear what you just received. As a general rule of thumb, only give the information when someone asks for it.

I cannot tell you how many times over the many years that I have heard "I get all kinds of intuitive hits as I work with my clients but I never tell them." If the person is with you as a client, then they have already decided to come to you for assistance. There is a myriad of reasons why practitioners do not share intuitive information with their clients. Here are some of the comments that I have heard:

"It is not my place to tell them what I saw. I just give massages."

"I think I am just making it up."

"I think they might get mad and never see me again."

"What if I am wrong?"

"It didn't make any sense to me so why should I tell them?"

"What if it doesn't make any sense to them?"

"If I share what I picked up it might make them feel bad today."

"I couldn't tell him during our session that I saw a spirit person standing behind him who had a message for him!"

Intuitive information continually bombards us. Do you sense the potentially rich information that is never shared? You do not need to be a professional healer or body worker to receive intuitive information for another.

Here is the distinction to be aware of. Only give intuitive information to people who have come to you as clients or those who simply ask you for intuitive information.

**Essential Point:**
*Do not surprise a person by giving them intuitive information that they did not ask for.*

Intuitive information is natural and everywhere, but it is pushed back, pushed down, and pushed away, never to be addressed. So many opportunities to learn from and so many opportunities to heal are right at the tip of awareness. We humans work so hard at keeping ourselves curtailed and smaller than we are naturally meant to be. Can you imagine the difference in life if we begin to share, with consideration of each individual, the richness of spirit information more openly?

**Receiving money or barter for the spiritual work you do.** People consistently ask me if it is all right to charge for spiritually based work. My response continues to be yes, absolutely. Spiritual people, offering spiritual assistance and insights to other spiritual people, also live in the material world. We need to pay our mortgage and buy gas and groceries just like the engineer who lives next door to us. No one questions other professions who are paid for their work and their insights. We too need to get paid because we too live in the material world.

I received a desperate email from a young woman who opened a retreat center that focused on Reiki. She was quite successful as an instructor of Reiki and she also drew in many people who received individual Reiki sessions from her. The desperate plea for help came when she could no longer pay the rent or purchase supplies for the center. She proudly informed me that spiritual practitioners should never charge for their services. "Healers are to serve Spirit and serve Reiki." She never charged for her services, her classes, or her knowledge because she was a healer. She is now floundering, confused, and bankrupt.

We are indeed spirits, dwelling in very material bodies, in a very material world, having a very material experience. It is all right for us to receive in the material experience. It is also all right with Spirit for us to flourish in this material experience. The woman who I just described is not working as a healer now because she did not allow herself to receive equal to all that she gave.

Money is simply a symbol of energy movement and a measurement of both our ability to give and our ability to receive. People acknowledge the value that your work has for them when they give you money for your services. Even more than that, it allows that person to complete the full cycle, the exchange of giving and receiving. "You have given to me and now I give back to you. We are complete."

Most of the world's societies base quality of life around money. Money seems to mean stability and freedom and, at the same time, evil and greed. Money is merely a symbol representing an individual's belief of their self-worth. When you align with the essence of your value and your worthiness, you will align with money. It is not evil. Money is only one example of an energetic symbol in the material world. Allow it to flow as you learn to flow with your soul. Receive equally to what you give. Receive now with grace.

# Chapter Two

# Can I Be a Medical Intuitive?

## Medical Intuition Is a Learned Skill

Stop right now!

Stop using negative terms for your intuitive abilities. You are not weird or odd. You are just perceiving the more complete world around you. Stop using terms such as weird, strange, odd, funny, or unusual as you discuss your perceptive realizations with others. More importantly, stop whispering those negative words, even to yourself, as life unfolds in new and surprising ways. You could be completely proud of your blossoming abilities. Instead of being blown away with a special synchronicity that just happened, begin now to expect magic to happen around you.

As you develop medical intuition, you will also become more cognizant of the natural mystical realm of life. It is simply a matter of expanding beyond the mundane thought processes in order to receive subtler nonphysical information around you. Begin to use only positive descriptive words for your developing abilities and take the negative words out of your experience. Use phrases such as:

"Of course that happened."

"I felt a deep knowing."

"I knew Spirit was with me when that happened."

"I listen to my intuition."

"I am intuitive."

"The spiritual world does exist."

Allow yourself to stand up straight with your eyes bright with pride, not dim with shame. Do not be ashamed that you sense and perceive more than those around you. They are only upset or afraid that they do not have the same understanding of life you obviously have.

**Essential Point:**
*Stop using negative terms about yourself and your intuitive abilities.*

The ability to sense and view the intimate story of another human is not magic and it is not a gift for the select few. It is a learned perception. We would not have to learn this skill if it had been treated as a natural acuity during our upbringing. We come into this life as sensitive organisms ready to take it all in! Slowly, we are told that our natural perceptions are wrong. What happens to us when our first grade teacher says the picture we drew of our dog is incorrect? "Dogs aren't purple. What color *should* your dog be?"

You are a little person trying to find information and answers about the world around you. Authority figures can be a teacher, an uncle, a parent, a minister, or any older person. You change your mind to appease them and then you change your drawing. Your dog no longer glimmers a translucent purple. You draw a black outline and fill it in with dark brown. Now you are matching your teacher's level of reality and beginning to forget the natural abilities you were born with.

Have you ever watched a new baby? They look all around the adults' heads. Most people think they are looking at their curly hair or the ceiling, but in reality, that baby is watching our aura shimmer and float around us. As the baby grows into an older child, he searches for ways to fit in with his superiors and our environment. As we grow older our natural, intense instincts are disregarded. We release the ability to pick up energetic information that we have been wired to perceive. We have not lost that ability. We have only forgotten to notice it.

Have you noticed that children up to the age of six or seven years old say the most spontaneous things? Things just gush out of their mouths. Inside of this gushing are remarkable insights and significant knowledge. One example is a child who constantly describes flying planes during the war and says that his real name is not what his parents keep calling him. When his parents researched this little boy's "imaginary name" and his "imaginary battles" and his death in combat, they found a man of that name who died as a fighter pilot. His parents were astounded and had to believe in their son's past life.

Another example happened in my own family. One of our children would cringe and hide behind something every time he heard a loud, unexpected sound. He would then explain he knew the sound was a plane dropping bombs on him. One of my grandchildren pointed to the back of her hand and told me that an angel came and kissed her right on that spot. Later on, that same little grandchild became irritated with her mother and said, "Don't you remember when I was the mommy and you were the little girl?"

Why don't we support our children and their awareness instead of smashing it out of them? Fear, you say? What are we afraid of? I believe we are terrified of our greatness, our bigness. We are afraid to be the co-creators of our universe. If each individual was allowed to be who they were meant to be, a tremendous momentum of creation would flourish on a much grander scale.

Fear diminishes our innate abilities. Many of us are afraid to be the creators we are meant to be. Our natural abilities for medical intuition are also stifled and smashed as we utter our first childhood words that do not fit into an adult's framework. When a child simply states that they have a little friend in the bedroom and the adult tells her that no one is there, the restrain and suppression begins. When a child in school draws his dog in purples and his teacher demands that he draw it in her reality, the smothering of his most instinctive, natural abilities continues. This has already happened to you in many, many ways throughout your life.

Your instinctive abilities are still there. You have only been trained and programed to ignore them! Once you realize this you can begin to "un-train" and re-train your mind and body and instincts. Yes, you can! Take your power back. If you continue to negate your natural abilities, you continue to give your power away. You are saying, "Adults in my life told me I was wrong so it must be true." You are the adult now. Take your power back and notice the entire world of the physical and, at the same time, the nonphysical.

I am a very clear medical intuitive because I do it every day in some manner. When I wake in the morning, I lie there for just a moment and ask someone for permission to look into their body and mind. As I go to sleep, I use that twilight time to check in on someone when they give me permission to do so. I include it within my working day, my day at home, my errand day. I practice, practice, and I practice some more. I am honing a skill. It is not magic or even a gift. It is an inborn, inherent function of humankind, and it is an inborn ability that you still have right now.

We are born with a natural psychic ability and we are able to use that ability to assist others with medical intuition. We are wired in a natural circuitry to send and receive energetic information. We are made to pick up sensitive signals from the environment around us and within us. Many people are already picking up medical intuitive information and not even realizing it. If they do notice it, they think they have no control over it. Yes you do, and yes you can!

**Essential point:**
*Our natural circuitry is wired to send and receive energetic information.*

Many people attending my medical intuitive workshop are professional intuitives already. Because much of the information comes from the energy field, the intuitive often does not access medical information because they are focusing on other topics for their client. Another world of information is available when they begin to include the intuitive information affecting the physical body.

Physicians, nurses, physical therapists, and other physical health practitioners naturally have a "knowing" in medical situations. They rely on instincts they have developed over years. For instance, a nurse can walk into the intensive care room and feel a change with her patient even before the bells and monitors go off. Healthcare workers in traditional settings are receiving medical intuitive information constantly, but most medically trained healthcare workers of all levels would never consider themselves a medical intuitive because they do not recognize their "instincts" as intuition.

Massage therapists, in the quiet darkness of their room, move easily into a place of knowing. As they work the body's muscles they begin to get into "the zone" where the thinking mind quiets and the universe of information flows in. At certain spots in the client's body, the massage therapist suddenly feels heartache or stress. The therapist then moves to a different area of the client's body and suddenly sees flashing images of the client fighting with her husband. In this "zone," the massage therapist naturally enters into the story of their client and understands where in the body the client is holding the emotions and thoughts, but even they do not identify themselves as medical intuitives.

**Three Primary Causes for Failing**

There are three primary causes for failing as a medical intuitive. They are fear, emotions, and expectations. Let's examine each reason for failure, one at a time, to assist you in recognizing your personal blockages and to rise out of that particular quagmire. Your excellence depends on distinguishing the methods of your failure because that understanding will free you from disappointment.

*1. Fear*

Fear is a sneaky beast. It comes in a myriad of shapes, sizes, degrees of severity, and modes. Fear has many disguises and is not always up front with you. It is difficult to identify because one moment it slaps you in the gut and the next moment it hides and lurks behind a screen of something else. For example, you might yearn to do medical intuition but something keeps getting in the way of putting this desire into action.

Deep inside you might be wondering if this training will change your life in some way. Change and the unknown future often terrifies people—the bigger the change, the bigger the fear and worry. Medical intuition might feel monumentally important to you. Here are some common fearful thoughts that might get into your way.

"If I learn this, what will my family think?"

"If I allow my intuition to develop, will it change my relationship with my partner?"

"What if I am successful with this? What will happen? Will I need to quit my job?"

"What if I try the medical intuitive class or learn from this book and I still cannot do it?"

"What do I do if I tell my client that she has an illness and she adamantly denies it?"

"I cannot stand being wrong in front of someone."

"I might fail at something again!"

Do you sense the potential underlying fear creeping around in your mind?

Many people are afraid of success. What if you are a clear and accurate medical intuitive? You might become well known and be in the spotlight. You have always had performance anxiety so you usually try to remain somewhat hidden from others.

Understand that success will work with you if you allow it to. Realize that you are in charge of the pace and rhythm of your life. The more you attune to the universal intelligence, the more delightfully successful you will become. The road, stretched out before you, becomes smoother and the old boulders become supportive gravel.

Increasing contact with the spirit realm is another fear. People worry that the more they are in contact with Spirit, the more they might be affected by the dark side. This saddens me. Heightening our inborn instincts and living with our innate skills will never plunge us into the dark. Expansion of the soul's true nature will always lead us toward the creation of life we are meant to live.

People used to have profound instincts when they lived in nature and lived from the land. We communicated with Spirit, the animal realm, and the land. We used to honor our inborn wisdom. Now, in our so-called advanced society, our instinctual, intuitive gifts are considered fearful. Receiving information from the universe brings us closer to the greatness of Source and the bigness that each of us are meant to be. The expansion of our awareness can only bring an expansion of life to us, not the dark.

Many people are afraid they will pick up illness or negative energy from the people they assist. You will not pick up or incorporate another's illness into your field. You will find yourself receiving the energy signals of stress and illness from another person during a session, but that is not the same as taking it on as your own.

### Essential point:
*When the session is over, you must not look back.*

When I feel a symptom of another person in my body, I command the following: "I thank you for this message. I will give it to my client. It is not mine. I release it now." I release the information from the reading and with a blessing, I release each person that I assist. It is up to them to live their own life with their own choices. I hope that they utilize the information that I give them, but I cannot make them. Allow yourself to deeply release each session to the point that you cannot remember a reading at the end of a day. People will ask you months later, "Don't you remember when you told me this?" No, I do not remember because I do not hold onto the energy of each person. You will not hold onto it either.

No matter how devastating or traumatic a situation is for that person, you must allow each person to have their own path, their own life, and their own responsibility. Focus completely on each person during the session, but when the session is over you must not look back. Release it and move back into your own life and your own energy.

Over and over again, I hear the same fear, not only from students but clients as well: "What if I am just making it all up?" People do not trust themselves, and so they do not trust the very spirit within their own body. Begin to accept, without exception, anything that instantly pops into your awareness and know it is correct on some level. Sometimes neither you nor your client will understand it immediately, but know that it is right.

**Essential Point:**
*Worrying about being right is the opposite of intuition.*

Take charge of your thoughts and know that fear is your outdated way of thinking. In fact, it might be someone else's fears and not even your own thinking. Most fears are learned from other people. What fears did you repeatedly hear from others as you grew up? Which fear did you learn and who did you learn them from? Did you learn to worry simply because your role model was a worrier or an "awful-izer"?

Decide that you are guiding your own thoughts now. You might find yourself thinking that you are failing again and again. This time, however, catch that old repetitive thought, jump behind the steering wheel of your life, and turn toward success. Every time you think that you are failing as a medical intuitive, catch yourself and consciously alter your thinking immediately. This is a process of discovery and awareness. Catch the fear and turn it around. Do this over and over and over again.

I was deep into a phone reading with a grief-stricken woman who had recently lost her husband. A giant snake unexpectedly rose up behind the woman's energetic form and hovered over her head. While it did not seem menacing in any way, it startled me nonetheless. I immediately decided not to tell her about this image because it seemed to have nothing to do with the topic at hand. I kept watching the persistent snake look at me from above her head, but I remained quiet about it because I thought my description of it would terrify her. My huge mistake! The very next thing that woman said was "Can you tell me why I am having snakes come up in all of my dreams lately?"

That is a true example of fear, not trusting my own abilities, and not trusting Spirit. I do this for a living and yet I sometimes "shoot myself in the foot" just like everyone else does. If at all possible, I don't want you to do this to yourself. Trust what pops into your mind and your vision for the person you are working with. It will always have value in some manner, even if it is a giant hovering snake!

Fear and worrying about being correct are the opposite of intuition. If you are concerned about being correct, you are in your thinking mind and not your intuitively aware mind. If you have any thoughts about self, you are not connecting psychically with the person you are trying to read for. If your thoughts are about worry or fear, then you have drifted far from your soul-self and far from your intent to assist someone. We cannot be in our spirit mind if we are in our thinking mind, especially if any of our thoughts are centered on self. Remember: worrying about being right is the opposite of intuition.

Anything that is fearful or limiting is not the voice of Spirit. There is no fear voiced or expressed through true Spirit. Fear only comes from the mind of humankind. Fear is not even known within the human body. The body, of its own accord, does not have fear. Fear is a specific thought energy that comes from within the mind and subsequently expresses through the physical human body. Spirit has no limits and never originates from fear. True, unaltered Spirit is all encompassing, all knowing, and exquisitely divine throughout all echelons of the cosmos.

**Essential Point:**
*Anything that is fearful or limiting is not the voice of Spirit.*

Document your impressions in your journal now.

### 2. Emotions

My eighteen-year-old cat Nicki began to show little interest in eating and as a result, she rapidly lost weight. One day, Nicki came over and sat on my lap, an unusual behavior for her. I placed my hands on her and instantly saw a tumor or a polyp flash through my mind's eye. I panicked and tried to go back and find its location. Nothing. I couldn't see a thing. I was too racked with emotion.

Our emotions will always hinder our intuitive success. If you are emotionally involved or invested in the reading, you will not receive accurate information. For example, excellent counselors never provide counseling for their own family members because it is impossible to grasp the intricacies of complicated family dynamics. The counselor has feelings about their own family that cloud their clinical perceptions.

Another example involves physicians. There is an unwritten understanding that a doctor never works on his or her own family or friends during critical situations. This unwritten rule exists because physicians are human and they cannot maintain an unobstructed clinical mind in an emergency when emotions are running high.

Why? Because humans cannot think and perceive clearly when they are emotional. People are in reaction mode and not a clear thinking mode. We are under a surge of stress hormones during an emotional event and that surge affects our ability to perceive and think clearly. We are not in our centered empowerment when we are reacting. I am the least precise when I am emotionally connected to the receiver of the reading, and you will not be precise either.

Emotions take energy and clarity away from intuition. Spirit information, more commonly called intuition, is usually neutral.

Rather than being full of emotion and opinion, Spirit neutrally offers guidance and neutrally stands back for each of us to make our choices. It is up to each person to be open and receptive to the guidance. We are the only thing that gets in our way, and we get in the way with thoughts that lead to beliefs that result in emotions. Emotional reactions wipe out the clarity of our intuition.

**Essential Point:**
*Emotions take energy and clarity away from intuition.*

You will often hear intuitives describe that they are at their best when they have never met the person before. Many intuitives even prefer phone readings because they do not see the individual personally. We are the most exact when we intellectually know the least about the person we are assisting. We must then rely on our innate intuitive instincts and not our thinking mind.

Here is a perfect example. My dearest friend of over forty years had been recently buried as I wrote this material in 2017. Had I attempted to give her family a reading right then, the swirling emotions inside of me would have obstructed my intuitive clarity. Even though my friend contacted me from the spirit realm and that contact was exceptionally pure, I still could not have been clear for my friend's family. Powerful emotions on my part would interfere with any spirit communications for them. Your clarity as a reader is vital for the client and vital for your own integrity.

Emotions are created from thoughts and beliefs. A belief is nothing more than a thought that we think frequently and have an emotional response to. Each emotion has an energetic signature. The deeper the emotion is felt, the more concrete and dense the energetic signature is. The longer that same emotion is held within, the more physical it becomes. It transforms into more substance and thus becomes more physical in nature.

Emotions are part of our natural makeup and expressing them in positive ways promotes health on every level. Emotions, when held inside and not expressed, drain energy from the body. That drain counteracts clear intent and clear intuition. Intent is a conscious focus of energy. It cannot take place when emotions are controlling your body and mind. Consider times in the past when you have noticed your personal emotions clouding your intent or your judgment.

Document your impressions in your journal now.

### 3. Expectations

And now for the grandest and most hidden blockage of all . . . our expectations! The Oxford Dictionary states an expectation is a strong belief that something will happen or be the case. It also describes expectation as a standard performance of something or someone. If we expect something to happen in a certain way and if that something happens in a different way, we will miss the truth of the event completely because we were focused on the expected outcome.

Expectations actually limit our perceptions of the world. An expectation is a strong thought that restricts all other possibilities. In fact, it confines our senses to the boundaries defined within the expectation. Our mind is not open to other prospects and thus we completely overlook the accurate information all around us. Intuitional information bombards us every minute of the day and night. If you think it must look a certain way or behave in a certain manner, vast dimensions of vital information are escaping you. If intuition does not come in the form or path you expect, then you are completely missing all the other pathways it is coming to you. This is a crucial point for success as a medical intuitive!

**Essential Point:**
*Expectations limit our perceptions of the world.*

Hundreds of thousands of people over the years have given up on their intuitive abilities because they were looking for something different than what was happening. Here is an example of one of the most common mistakes people make. If you think intuitive information will appear visually, as a solid image, and you are only noticing a strange metallic smell, you will think that you are not getting any intuitive information. In fact, you will disavow the smell and not even consider it as information. In this example, ignoring a strange smell literally means that you completely missed an important piece of information for your client. That strange metallic smell might have been an intuitive signal that your client is toxic from heavy metal poisoning from working in a laboratory for the last fifteen years.

If you have it in your mind that medical intuition will come to you in a certain manner, you have set your intent to notice intuition through only one pathway. You have eliminated all other modes of perception by trying so hard to perceive in only one certain way. Release all expectations. Be thrilled that you never know what is going to happen next when you sit for a reading. Be there for the full adventure of it. Set your intent to receive the entire story in any form that it presents itself.

**Essential Point:**
*If you expect intuition to come in one particular way, you are missing all the ways it is truly coming to you.*

Trust, trust, and trust some more. When you trust your intuition you are really trusting Spirit and trusting your own soul. This is worth repeating. When you trust your intuition you are really trusting Spirit and trusting your own soul. Take charge of this and know that you are in control of you. Completely align with self-trust. As you do this you will notice the sensation of honor. Have you ever honored someone else? Honor is assessing and recognizing a profound treasured value. Give this to yourself now. Honoring has a certain physical sensation within. You can recreate that feeling within your own physical body right now as you trust and honor the empowered greatness within you.

As you consider the three primary blockages of fear, emotion, and expectations, allow yourself to honestly evaluate which one affects you the most or which one occasionally raises its ugly head and gets in your way. Honesty about yourself at this point is crucial to your success. Allowing random thoughts to have control of your mind will always hinder your development toward your intuitive goals. Begin to first search for your particular mode of failure or the combination of ways to fail. Be honest with your thoughts and emotions. Evaluate how your expectations regarding intuitive phenomena have blinded you to the uncountable avenues through which Spirit has been communicating with you.

**Essential Point:**
*Honesty about yourself at this point is crucial to your success.*

Simply be aware how your particular blockage presents itself and what happens to you when it rises up. Take your time as you notice and learn about yourself. Be aware of all the ways you have not been in charge of yourself.

Document your impressions in your journal now.

### You Are Not the Only One Afraid

The medical intuitive is not the only one with fear. The person about to receive your intuitive assessment is fearful too. This might be their first time to receive a reading and they do not know what to expect. Their thoughts might be racing:

"What if she tells me when I am going to die? Do I want to know that?"

"What if this person tells me I have cancer?"

"What do I do if she tells me that my spouse is having an affair? Can I take it?"

"What if the psychic says I will get into a car wreck?"

The fearful thoughts go on and on because, at some level, the client knows you are accessing the full story of their life—the good, the bad, and the ugly.

As my phone session began, I saw a human form that was

neither male nor female. As soon as I focused on the form, it ran away! I refocused and tried to bring the human form back into my "viewing area." Three times the human energetic form ran away. I stopped trying to connect intuitively and simply discussed my experience with my client in that moment. She immediately agreed that she was fearful about the reading. She hesitantly said that it felt deeply invasive to her because she was so surprised by my accuracy. We discussed this and she quickly realized that this hesitancy, and the feeling that her privacy was being invaded, became very important information about her life struggles. Hiding from her fears and how I perceived her running away became the focus of the reading.

On another occasion, I saw the client's energetic form hiding under a big blanket, peeking out once in a while like a frightened but fascinated child. She, too, identified a sense of fear about receiving a reading and what secrets might be revealed. She was afraid but excited at the same time. At the end of the session, this woman told me that she could feel a dramatic change in her body and mind.

At the beginning of both readings, I thought something was wrong with me. Maybe I was too tired or too distracted to do the reading. Then I quickly followed my own advice, thank goodness, and simply told the person what I was picking up, what it looked like, and how it felt like fear. They both heartily agreed and the rest of the reading went on from there.

Let your client know when you pick up fear and discomfort. Allow your perceptions regarding their fear to become part of your reading. Honestly tell your client what you perceive about their fearfulness. That fear will become part of the session. Discussing it will lead the client to understand how fear is interfering in their life.

As a medical intuitive practitioner, you will tap into portions of your client's eternal story. Our individual story consists of all the traumas and all the emotions of shame and guilt, and the agony of grief. A fearful mind is in protection mode. It will always try to protect its person in whatever way it can. Notice how protection presents itself with each person and include it as part of your reading. If someone's fear comes up with you during a session, you can expect that fear will also show up in other areas of their lives.

The medical intuitive, under all circumstances, must create an ambiance of comfort, security, and hope. Never take hope away. I never inform someone about their death or the death of a loved one even when I am clearly perceiving it. You might find yourself talking about death with your client in surprising ways. For example, I found myself visualizing a past life for one gentleman. I told him that he was walking down a street in London sometime in the 1800s. As evening came, he slowly turned a corner and walked into a deserted alley. He leaned against a brick wall and collapsed on the pavement. He quickly died of a heart attack.

I described the ease with which he passed and his readiness for the transition. The distinct past life images and sensations that I saw generated a long discussion about death. My client explored his feelings about death with me for quite some time and at the end of the session he thanked me for discussing the matter with him.

About a month later another client came in for a session. Out of the blue she asked me if I knew the client who had died of a heart attack in a previous life. I told her that I was very confidential for my clients and denied any knowledge of this man. She said, "Oh, for some reason I thought you knew him, so I wanted you to know he died a few weeks ago." While outwardly I kept my counselor composure, I was stunned. Had Spirit guided my intuitive impressions and led me to discuss death with him? Was he supposed to be in my office to help him prepare for his imminent death in the next week? The ways of Spirit are remarkable. We only need to get our intellectual mind out of Spirit's way and out of our own way.

While I never predict death, I do offer warnings of danger and give guidance about alternatives. For example, I informed a man that he suffered from extremely high blood pressure. At the same time I saw him walking and exercising more. I saw him walking quite slowly at first and then walking faster as he built up strength. He responded by telling me that he used to walk every day and his blood pressure decreased when he did so. This man received a medical warning but also a healing action to take. I let him know that I could see positive results for him as he made the choice to heal.

Give your client the energy of caring compassion *and* give them the factual information that you pick up. Offer them insights about taking charge of their mind and body, and guide them toward the myriad of choices in life. I receive a great deal of information about options clients can do to begin their healing process. I never recommend that they stop traditional medical treatment, instead using the information from my assessment in conjunction with their current medical treatments.

# Chapter Three

## It's All Electrical

### We Humans Are Powerful

Have you ever wondered why we medical practitioners, healers, and bodyworkers are even needed to step in and assist our clients in the first place? Why are people not healing themselves, on their own? Why does it take others to assist in the healing process? I have two thoughts about these questions.

My first thought is that we humans are not meant to live our lives as an island. We are meant to share this earth experience together. We each are meant to contribute to each other's experience in either a positive way or what we humans might think of as a negative way. We have choices in how we participate in this massive system of the Universe.

It took me years to realize the second answer. We are powerful because we are human. We are meant to be powerful because we are a vital link in the system of the cosmos. We are not meant to be the weakest link. We are not meant to be victims of the system. We are meant to own our empowerment and utilize it for each other. Feel and understand that you and I and every human on this earth are key components, not only for ourselves but in the lives of others as well.

This is why the non-physical world responds so readily for us. When we call out to the non-physical realms of our guides, angels, and healing beings, they respond. This explains why they will not interfere in our lives without our request. It is not because we are weak. It is because we are a link in the structure and the organization of the Universe that is just as powerful as all the other beings within it.

We are creators. Our brain functions as a computer. Our mind, however, is everywhere. I will repeat that. Our mind is everywhere. It is our aliveness. It is in each and every physical cell of our physical body. It emanates beyond our skin and is commonly known as the aura. It is within our soul and it makes up our soul. The mind is the internet with a natural access to the world within you, the material world around you, and the infinite world beyond this world.

Energy is electrical in nature, vibrating at certain frequencies. Each and every frequency holds informational signatures within it. Everything is energy, and energy is information. The human body and brain are receivers and senders of energy. We humans are vibrating electrical forms living within an electrically vibrating world.

Gary Schwartz, PhD, in *The Living Energy Universe: A Fundamental Discovery that Transforms Science and Medicine,* stated, "Remember, information and energy continuously span out into space, and like lightening, the info-energy that actually precedes us is traveling close to the speed of light. This means that the information and energy arrives much sooner than the physical system does. Our electromagnetic signals always precede us."

Each and every thought and subsequent emotion is also vibrating electrical energy forms rushing from brain to body and back to the brain and back to the body in a continual flood of information. For example, thoughts of worry have an energy signature that is slow and sluggish. That dense energy floods your body every time you have that particular worry. If you worried about something ten times today, each wave of that particular vibration builds on the last one, congealing and becoming thicker and denser. This thickness of thought and emotion actually creates more and more "weight" and, if you continue worrying all day, every day, it develops substance. This thickening substance can literally form and congregate in your body, eventually forming an illness of some type. Just think what might happen if you feel deep fear, anxiety, or guilt for long periods of time!

We are truly creators. Think of the magnitude of that! If we can alter non-physical energy into an illness, what on earth might we be capable of doing with positive, loving thought energy? The most significant and powerful concept I will say in this book is this: We are already creators on the most subtle yet most important level of all—energy.

Candace Pert, in *Everything You Need to Know to Feel Good*, stated this concept in her words: "Besides receiving and processing information to unify a single bodymind, the peptides and receptors are clumped to form ion channels to pump ions in and out of the cell. This rhythmic, pulsating movement creates an electrical current that meanders through the body, influencing the state of excitability or relaxation of the entire organism."

Pert also noted that the chakra centers based along the spine appear to have a concentrated level of these "molecules of emotions," thus creating energetic and chemical intake and output centers for processing information. Here again is confirmation that the ethereal wisdom of the East and the allopathic research of the West continue to merge in the natural expansion of knowledge.

According to Rollin McCraty, Director of Research for the Institute of HeartMath, the heart is more involved in this bodymind than we could have ever guessed. It is much more than the pump that pushes blood around. The heart not only pushes blood around, but it also sends out electrical frequencies that resonate with the brain's rhythms and interacts with the earth's electromagnetic field. The Institute of HeartMath has measured the electrical field of the human heart and found that it radiates far beyond the body. This prestigious organization has found that our heart energy literally interconnects us with other people as well as with animals and the earth.

And if you think all this is amazing, wait until you read this! The heart has cells that are exactly like some of the cells in our brains. Yes, our hearts have brain cells. According to the Institute of HeartMath, as electrical pulses move back and forth between the heart and the brain, the heart sends more information to the brain than the brain does to the heart. Our hearts have brain power. I love this kind of information!

Here are some other findings from the Institute of HeartMath:

- The quality of our thoughts and emotions affect the heart's electromagnetic field. The HeartMath Institute works to confirm the theory that our negative and our positive thoughts affect our heart.

- The heart has short- and long-term memory. Are you aware that heart transplant recipients frequently report having different thoughts, habits, and cravings after their transplant? The changes have been found to fit the personality of the heart donor!

- The heart is sensitive to the magnetic fields of the earth. Our intentional thoughts affect the earth.

- The heart sends out smooth rhythms when a person feels emotions such as appreciation. Those rhythms become jagged and chaotic when that same person feels frustration.

- The heart generates oxytocin, which is the "feel good hormone." Prior to this finding, it was thought that only the brain generated this hormone.

We have heart intelligence. Let's use it in profound ways.

Air and space is also full of throbbing energy. We already know that radio waves, cell phone waves, television signals, and satellites fill the atmosphere around us. It is said that there is more empty space in outer space than there are planets and stars. My human anatomy books also state there is more space around each cell in our body than there are cells. Can you see where I am going with this?

The space within us is not empty and the space around us is not empty. According to a program presented on the PBS television show *Nova*, "Empty space is not empty. It is flooded with activity

. . . Space is expanding and accelerating." This episode, based on the book *Fabric of the Cosmos: Space, Time and the Texture of Reality* by Brian Greene, goes on to say that something now called spacetime is like stretchy fabric that is never static but rather is dynamic and very active. Space is now considered flexible, and time is flexible. This unseen, empty space makes up 70 percent of the Universe.

The space between you and the moon and beyond the moon is an undulating, throbbing world of aliveness that is heaving with electrical information. Everything in the Universe spins, has cycles and rhythms. Everything in our experience is cyclical and flows in rhythms. It is as if the cosmos throb like a heartbeat of traveling energy, pulsating in wave-like patterns. The entire intergalactic system is a generator.

Gary Schwartz, in *The Energy Healing Experiments*, stated it this way: "I learned that human beings actually are antennas. Wherever we go, whatever we do, we silently and invisibly pick up radio and TV signals—and numerous other electromagnetic frequencies—just like rabbit-ears antenna."

Electrolytes within the human body also play a vital role in the cosmic electrical system. By definition, these electrolytes are sodium, potassium, magnesium, calcium, and chloride, which are substances whose aqueous solutions conduct electricity. Look at a map of the Earth's surface and you will see that most of the globe's surface is water. According to the United States Geological Survey, 70 percent of the earth's surface is water and 97 percent of the water is salt water. Salt water is a great conductor of electricity. The entire globe is a giant conductor for electromagnetic energy.

Electrolytes are essential elements within the electrical system of the physical body. When they are not at a healthy level, the electrical system begins to break down. We cannot think because the signals do not reach the brain properly, and the brain cannot process the electrical signals that do arrive. The heart depends on the electrolytes to maintain its beat and the contraction of its muscles. The electrolytes in the body are the same elements that make up the earth. The earth is in our bodies and we are a part of the earth. Throw in some water and voila, flowing electricity!

Richard Gerber, MD, stated in *Vibrational Medicine*: "In metaphysical literature, this energy field that surrounds and penetrates living systems is referred to as the 'etheric body.' It is said that the etheric body is one of many bodies contributing to the final expression of the human form. The etheric body, in all likelihood, is an energy interference pattern similar to a hologram . . . Perhaps the universe itself is a gigantic 'cosmic hologram.' That is to say, the universe is a tremendous energy interference pattern. By virtue of its likely holographic characteristics, every piece of the universe not only contains but also contributes to the information of the whole. The cosmic hologram is less like a holographic still photo frozen in time than it is like a holographic videotape dynamically changing from moment to moment."

You and every other human are co-creators with the entire Universe. We are taking part in a developing and changing video of development. Consciousness, like the Universe, never stands still. It has energy and is always moving, creating, and expanding. The development of each individual person sends information into the universal collective, which in turn intensifies the energetic momentum and expands the consciousness of the All. We are washed in a bath of vibrational information.

Now some thoughts about the aura, which manifests as a particular kind of electric energy.

The aura is made up of every thought and emotion that we have ever experienced. It holds our secrets, our beliefs, our fears, our past, and our potential. The past can be five minutes ago or five thousand years ago. The visible aura is a portion of our awareness shimmering beyond the edges of the body. It is a combination of thought, emotion, and physical sensation in the vessel of a human body. When you witness the aura you are actually seeing the soul.

Dr. Gary Schwartz, stated in his book, *The Living Energy Universe*: "Information has energy, and energy has information. Information without energy is 'powerless'; energy without information is 'purposeless.' Together they are quite a team. Soul and spirit are also quite a team. Could it be that soul is to spirit as information is to energy?"

Dr. Schwartz goes on to say: "Recall that energy is power and information is system—when we view them both as dynamic and interactive processes, we logically come to a new, living vision of energy and information, spirit and soul—the living energy universe."

In *Physics of the Soul*, Amit Goswami, PhD, stated: "They [souls] carry the conditioning and the learning of previous incarnations, but they cannot add to or subtract from the conditioning by further creative endeavors, which can be done only in conjunction with earthly form. The reason is subtle."

### Essential Point:
*Notice each person as an energetic soul.*

Imagine seeing or meeting each and every person first as a pulsating electrical energetic soul. Notice the soul of someone that you do not know. Notice the soul of someone who is not acting right. Notice the soul of someone that you know. Notice the soul of someone who lives and thinks differently from you. Notice the soul of someone who has hurt you.

Describe your awareness in your journal now.

## Thoughts, Emotions, Illness, and Allowing

As mentioned earlier, the molecules in your body are vibrating in hundreds of melodies and harmonies, all of them performing simultaneously. What happens when illness takes place? What happens when we get something as simple as the common cold, a stubbed toe, or an earache? What is going on when someone receives the diagnosis of cancer or multiple sclerosis?

In the 1930s a researcher named Harold Burr began an in-depth study of cancer in mice. His study was different than most. The abstract entitled "Harold Burr's Biofields: Measuring the Electromagnetics of Life, summarized by Ronald E. Matthews, M.S." describes how Burr measured the energy field of mice before and after they were injected with cancer. He discovered that the energy around the chest of a mouse increased by several thousand microvolts ten to fourteen days before there was any evidence of a tumor. The energy level began to fluctuate from the normal levels before the physical body showed any evidence of cancer. This was groundbreaking science for the 1930s, but it did not influence the medical world of today.

The body, mind, and emotional connection is real. We can learn all types of information if we begin to listen to the signals. For example, consider the vibrational signal of a stubbed toe. What pops into your mind regarding a stubbed toe? You might be worried about taking a tiny step in a new direction today. You may already feel that a decision you made this morning just doesn't feel right or you might have just felt irritated at your spouse an hour ago and now you are even more irritated about this painful toe.

Another simple example of receiving energetic messages might be the earache your friend had last week. Often the cause of an earache is inflammation somewhere in the inner ear. Notice if your friend has complained about the sound of a co-worker's screechy voice or their children making too much noise. An earache may be the result of those thoughts and emotions.

Begin to listen to the signals of your body before the symptoms of illness become manifest. What do people usually do when they are not heard? They become much louder. The signals of illness will also become louder. The symptoms will build and build in an attempt to be recognized.

I often hear people say during a reading that a chakra center in someone's body is closed. While that might be the case, it seems more probable that the center is struggling with resistance. People struggle with resistance and struggle to control life. We often try to get people to change so that we are more comfortable. We want our spouse to be different; our children to be different; our family members to be different than they really are. We often want to be different as well.

Notice the language that people use. We fight against cancer and other religions. We have the war on drugs and the war on terror. We are warriors against this and that. Fighting against something, no matter what it is, actually builds up the energy of the thing you are fighting against. Resistance and fighting creates a heavy, forceful, and jarring vibration.

When we continue to resist something, that resistance eventually happens within the human body in various degrees of illness. For example, resistance can be caused by something like feeling worried to take a tiny new step in life or it can be as profound as something eating away at you for thirty years. Resistance against something creates more restriction. If there is a kink in your garden hose, the flow of water is stifled. If there is war going on within you and the war continues on and on, the resistance builds. The body you inhabit right now interacts and participates with your thoughts, with your emotions, and with the entire universe where you dwell.

**Essential Point:**
*Resistance against something creates more restriction.*

As we consider resistance, I ask you to consider the meaning of the word "allow." I have found that the word "allow" creates more powerful reactions in people than resistance does. Why? Because most people do not want to allow others just to be who they are. Most people struggle to allow life to unfold just as it is. For some, allowing means laziness, and for others it means selfishness, self-centeredness, or hardened callousness. So people continue to fight the great fight because we have been trained to do it that way. We receive more accolades and awards in battle than we do in peace, but our physical bodies take the brunt of the battle. The resistance grows heavy over the years, creating illness and disease over time.

I am not asking you to sit on the couch for the remainder of your life and never take any action. I am asking you to consider feeling the flow of your own life and the flow of every human around you. Your family's and friends' flows might appear wildly different from your own. Please notice right now the profound struggle or heartache or fear that difference may be causing you.

Your life choices and interests might also be scaring your family and friends. One of the greatest obstacles I hear in my workshops involves how family and friends might respond to someone's interest in medical intuition:

"My family would be so upset if they knew I was learning medical intuition right now in your workshop."

"I just know that my friends would leave me if they found out about the level of my intuitive abilities."

Please begin to *allow*. Allow them their life's path and please continue on with your life's path. I am asking you to take right action in your own life. Take action that feels deeply comfortable and smooth in the depth of your gut. The more you live your truth and live your dreams, the healthier, happier, and wiser you become.

### Essential Point:
*The more you live your truth and live your dreams,*
*the healthier, happier, and wiser you become.*

Life is an intricately complex set of thoughts, feelings, circumstances, and experiences. That complex combination lives and breathes with wisdom beyond human understanding. You can succumb to its intensity in disease or you can flow with its vital force. When you understand that life is about the exploration, the fascination, and the expansion of awareness, your body responds with a fine, buoyant energy that vibrates the human body toward healing.

# PART TWO

## Prepare to Excel as a
## Medical Intuitive

# Chapter Four

## Prepare Your Thoughts and Mind

### Imagination, Intuition, and Day Dreaming

Intuition is the ability to harvest information that is presented to us in both non-physical and physical form. Intuition consists of non-physical wave lengths of data that come to us from all directions. For example, I was once sitting in my car at a busy intersection contemplating an issue in my life. I closed my eyes for a few seconds and asked Spirit for direct guidance that I would not be able to miss. Just as I opened my eyes, a large truck flew through the intersection with one word painted in giant letters across the truck. It was exactly what I was hoping for and it was the answer to my dilemma! Intuitive information is absolutely everywhere if only we allow ourselves to notice.

Intuition will always seem and feel like your imagination. I will repeat that. It will *always* feel like your imagination. Intuition makes contact with us through our sensory mind and not the thinking mind. While spirit information is non-physical in nature, Spirit also utilizes the physical world around us. Intuition has nothing to do with our educational level or life experience. We can choose to receive it or not.

The left side of the human brain is geared for detailed, logical material such as analyzing statistics, reconciling your checkbook, reading text books, and memorizing material. The right side of the brain is wired for concepts and feelings, and sensing the bigger picture of life and experiences. The right hemisphere captures and processes images and sensory experiences. It is the area that lights up when we are creative and using our imagination. The right hemisphere is also the receiving center and the processing center of non-physical intuitive information.

## Essential point:
### *Intuition will always feel like your imagination.*

Imagination is the voice and wavelength of non-physical information. Imagination, from Webster's Dictionary, means "the act or power of forming a mental image of something not present to the senses or never before wholly perceived in reality." This definition does not say that it is fallacy.

My hero Albert Einstein had an observation about imagination: "The true sign of intelligence is not knowledge but imagination." How profound for a genius, famous for his thoughts, to recognize that the thinking mind is not the entire story! We cannot do our intuitive work without imagination. Assume from this moment forward that you will be utilizing your imagination. Stop trying to discount it or push it away. Imagination must now be your companion.

Imagination is the electrical current that infinite intelligence rides upon. The greater consciousness of the cosmos flows to you in the form of intuition. This accumulated consciousness contains the wonder and marvels of all that has been achieved and all that has been realized. I repeat again—your intuition will *always* seem as if you are making it up. It will *always* seem like imagination because it is an electrical current of powerful, intelligent communication.

## Essential Point:
### *We cannot do our intuitive work without imagination.*

Did you know that intuitive information will not be wrong? Whether you receive information for yourself or for another, there is truth in it on some level. Can you imagine that all intuitive information is accurate and has meaning on some level? You may not understand it at the moment because it comes from many levels and planes of accumulated intelligence from all that has been and all that is possible, from the physical and the non-physical realms.

It is the interpretation of information that gets us into trouble. If you are receiving intuitive information about yourself, then by all means interpret away. But if you are working with another person, refrain from interpreting or trying to explain the insights that you are receiving. When you begin to interpret intuitive information for another, you interject your personal experience into theirs.

**Essential Point:**
*Interpret intuition for yourself but do not*
*interpret for another.*

Interpretations come from your thinking mind as it tries to make sense of an image, a word, a phrase, or a symbol for another person. You and the person you are working with are two drastically different people. The thinking mind is not able to interpret intuitive information you receive for other people because the thinking mind is more about our personal life experience and not the life experience of another.

For example, if I see a snake rising upward during a medical intuitive scan, and I love snakes, my interpretation would probably reflect that love. My client, however, might understand it as a life-threatening experience with a poisonous snake in his childhood. As a result, that fear is locked in his abdomen and, even now as a forty-year-old adult, it continues to create severe, unexplained stomach pain. He has gone through medical test after medical test and each time the physicians insist that nothing is wrong.

Can you tell that the accuracy of my information could possibly be damaged because of my personal interpretation? If I had told this man that I see a snake and it means love, that man would not be able to adjust his visceral reaction to realize that my impression of a snake was profoundly accurate. He might possibly evaluate my reading as farfetched and give me no credit for the evidence I revealed. As a result, healing, centered on an interpretation, would probably not happen.

If I, however, simply informed the client that I perceive the symbol of a snake rising up from his abdomen, he will know exactly what it is about and he will also know that I had an amazing ability to assist him to heal that old childhood experience.

That meditative, daydream zone where we go to imagine is built right into our system like a computer program. When we slide into that daydream time we are gathering and assimilating information from the last two hours of life. As we assimilate the information within our mind and brain, we also upload the information to the collective consciousness of the cosmos. This daydreamlike brain wave state is also how we download information from the greater collective intelligence. We call that download intuition.

The daydreamlike, meditative brain wave essentially transfers us from the left brain of worldly details to the right brain activities of intuitive knowledge. In other words, our chatty, controlling left brain is not in charge. The noise of the thinking mind subsides and we have a chance to truly get out of our own way. Intuitive information is not about thinking, thinking, and thinking some more. It is about sensing, sensing, and sensing even more.

Let's discuss daydreaming in general to prepare you to practice with the following individual steps. Recall the sensation of daydreaming. Remember where you usually sit when you slide into a daydream space. Remember how gentle it feels. It does have a certain feel to it. Your mind and your body know exactly all the sensations of going into the "zone."

**Essential Point:**
*Concentration will never increase your psychic abilities.*

Your thoughts and your body slip quietly aside as the daydream creates itself. You are not in the forefront of your mind because the daydream sensations move into the forefront. You feel somewhat hazy, vague, and dreamlike. You are not thinking. In fact, there are few thoughts, and each thought feels softer than the one just a moment ago. You suddenly become more visual and your daydream comes in images and bodily sensations. You have more distinct sensations and more distinct feelings. Your daydream is far from being numb or unaware. You are actually in a heightened state of awareness that is not dependent or involved with your intellect. Notice the distinctive nature of it.

As you feel the daydreamlike state of being, you are tuning into a finer vibration of energy. You are leaving the mundane earth vibration and moving upward and outward. This will allow thought energy from other realms to enter into your awareness. You have opened your energy to receive and include telepathic awareness. Accept the most instant, the most immediate information in the myriad of ways that it might come to you.

You absolutely know this state of being. It is a natural rhythm for the human brain. It comes naturally throughout the day, but you can also cause your mind to go to this rhythm. No one can make you do this and no one can do it for you. You are the only one who knows the impressions and sensations of your dreamy space and place. You can send yourself into that state of being at will when you choose. You simply direct your mind to do this on command.

**Telepathy or Our Thinking Mind?**

Telepathy seems to be the most unrecognized path to receive intuitive information from the Universe, another living person, or a person in spirit. Telepathy can happen purposely or it can be picked up randomly anywhere from the energy field. Since thought is energy, it can be projected toward us and we can project thought energy outward to others. We can also merge with thought energy and enter into its field. Thought energy can also accumulate in or around our energy field.

**Essential Point:**
*Do not search for intuitive information. Take only
what pops into your awareness.*

Those of you who are deliberately working to enhance your intuitive abilities often are confused between your logical thinking mind and your telepathy. In that confusion, everything seems like your thinking mind and nothing else. Telepathic information is completely obliterated in that confusion. One of your most important intuitive pathways comes through thoughts.

### Essential Point:
*There is no effort to send and receive*
*telepathic information.*

Telepathy is a major pathway by which we humans receive information. It is not the same as our logical thinking mind. It is our natural ability to receive and send informational waves. The key to recognizing telepathy is to notice that there is no effort in this transference of information back and forth. Your thinking mind did not have time to get in the way because telepathic information comes in so quickly. It is instantaneous.

If you feel like you are searching in your mind for intuitive information, you are putting forth too much effort. If you find yourself searching or trying hard to receive intuitive impressions, you are in your thinking mind and this will completely block your telepathic pathway.

### Essential Point:
*Trust the instant thought or image and ignore the next.*

This is important to note. Telepathy is how our spirit guides speak to us. It is the most active pathway to inform us about our own life, and it is how they inform us regarding our clients too. The clearest intuitive information will always pop, jump, leap, or dart into our awareness and feel as if it came out of nowhere.

Trust what you get with absolute confidence. In other words, allow yourself to receive information and do not alter it in any way. Your logical thinking mind will hinder you if you allow it to. If you tend to be critical, then critical thoughts will try to get in your way. If you tend to censor your words for the sake of others, then that type of thought will get in your way as well.

The following case study is an example of the level of self-trust you must have and you must maintain.

I always liked working with Linda and her energy because she was so attentive and interested in learning and discovering more about herself. What I especially adored about her was how she applied what she learned. This kind of introspection endeared me to her.

During one of her sessions, enormous bubbles rose up from the top of Linda's head. It seemed quite dramatic due to the size of the leak and the speed at which it was gushing from the top of her head, slightly to the left of center. I sent energy for a long period of time into that spot. After ten minutes or so, the bubbles slowed and then finally stopped. I informed her about this and she adamantly said that nothing had happened to her head. I probably looked as confused as I felt. I told Linda that something very traumatic must have happened, but she insisted that nothing had. As I continued with the rest of my reading, her eyes suddenly lit up and she exclaimed, "Oh, wait a minute! When I was at work, I rose up under my machine and hit my head. I about knocked myself out and I was covered in blood. I had a large bump and a cut in my skull. Maybe I should have gotten stitches."

A few years later Linda offered another interesting situation. She asked me to take a look at her foot and especially her little toe. A great deal of pain released from the toe, and when I took a closer look psychically, I could see a complete break across the base of her toe. When I told her about the break she said she did go to the emergency room, but the x-ray did not show any broken bones. I told her that it was definitely broken and to tape it to the toe next to it to give it some stability as it continued to heal. Linda said okay but reminded me again that it was not broken. She returned about a month later and told me that a follow-up x-ray had in fact showed a broken bone in her toe exactly as I had seen it!

In the first example, Linda did not remember the injury to her head and adamantly denied that anything could have caused the "leak." I could have decided right then and there that I was terrible at this "psychic stuff" and stopped developing my medical intuition because of it. In the second situation, an x-ray confirmed that my psychic perceptions of her broken toe were exactly correct! I was completely confident in both episodes that my perceptions were clear and accurate, and I did not change my impressions to fit the client's responses. I trust myself and I trust Spirit.

Inform the person of images, physical sensations, smells, sounds, telepathic thoughts and waves of knowing that simply flood your awareness. Most important, you must trust yourself and your psychic instincts without hesitation.

The ability to distinguish the difference between your own internal thoughts and intuitive information is imperative. Do not search for intuitive information. Always accept that initial pop of intuitive information. Send your mind into the daydreamlike brain wave, pause, and accept the first thing that jumps into your awareness.

## Meditation Made Simple

Meditation stills the thinking mind and at the same time allows the spirit mind to expand and experience more. Meditation allows the electromagnetic frequency of the spirit mind to expand and link with the electromagnetic vibration of Source. Meditation is an absolute necessity in fostering medical intuitive skills. You cannot access the realm of spirit if your brain remains consumed in physical experiences, physical objects, and physical distractions. Meditation unifies and expands our brain wave energy to create an intermingling with Source. It is an absolute requirement for our medical intuitive development.

*There are three primary secrets for successful meditation.*

**Secret 1:** Never fight against your thoughts for you will never win. You must stop the battle immediately and call a truce with your thoughts. The next step is to make friends with your thoughts and simply watch them as spurts and surges of energy. Have you ever considered your thoughts as spurts and surges of energy? Positive thoughts flow in a finer, tighter frequency, while negative thoughts surge in a wider, thicker, and heavier band of energy.

As you consider watching your thoughts, you will at first have a habit of watching the topic of each thought. As you continue to notice the topic of each thought, you can begin to notice them in yet a different manner. As you watch your personal thoughts, notice each of them more as spurts or even surges of energy. Some move quite rapidly and some thoughts move gently. Notice that you are not attempting to stop your thoughts but in fact are deepening your awareness of them and allowing them to continue to flow in and by. As the flow continues, watch and feel it as a fascinated, not frustrated, observer. Feel the difference?

**Secret 2:** Shorten the time that you sit in meditation. Most people who are new to meditating try to sit for half an hour or even a full hour. They become restless and easily distracted and sense their failure as a result. People cannot go from their hectic, over-stimulated day, then suddenly sit down and expect to slide into a different consciousness for long periods of time.

As beginners, we need to take it more slowly, more gently, and more lovingly. Give yourself some time to slow down and just begin to think about meditating and how you will be doing it in the next few minutes. Thinking about meditating for a few minutes will give your brain time to adjust from frenzied activity to a calmer, quieter experience. Then, when you sit down to actually meditate, your body and mind have had a chance to acclimate to the experience. This is key. Sit for only three to five minutes at a time. Anything more is too long. If you try to push beyond five minutes you are setting yourself up for failure.

Most books on meditation ask that you set aside a time to meditate and those same books ask you to create a space in your home, usually with an altar, that is your meditation space. If you have been able to do that and it is working for you, then for goodness' sake, continue to do that for yourself. If, however, you never find yourself in that space or have not even created that space, here is a different idea: incorporate meditation into your day, wherever you are and whatever you are doing.

Incorporate meditation throughout your daily life. Look for three-minute segments within your day. When do those three-minute segments occur? You might realize that booting up your computer takes a few minutes. It takes a few minutes when you get caught by that long train on the way to work. You might realize that you stand in the grocery line even longer than five minutes, and what about waiting in the doctor's office? Have you noticed that when you awake in the morning you usually lie there for a few minutes?

Bring meditation into your life today and incorporate it into your personal rhythm.

**Essential Point:**
*Never fight against your thoughts for you will never win.*

Here are some easy steps to guide you into meditation. Read through all of these steps first to get a sense of it. I also offer an audio version on my website to assist you in meditation. If you are a beginner, only meditate for three minutes per sitting.

**Simple Meditation Steps**

1. Be physically comfortable as you sit and do not lie down. If you are incorporating meditation into your day, be comfortable even if you are standing. Do not cross arms or legs. Relax and consciously lower your shoulders. Allow your teeth to part a little and let your jaw find its resting place. The tip of your tongue will rest naturally on the roof of your mouth.

2. Slightly move your head around until you feel it naturally balanced atop your spine.

3. Close your eyes or let your eyelids partially close.

4. Allow your eyes to gently roll upward. Do not push or force your eyes. Let it be a gentle feel of looking slightly upward.

5. Welcome all thoughts and do not fight against your thoughts. Remember—if you battle, you will lose the battle. Thoughts are not the enemy unless you make them that way. Let your thoughts rush in if they want. Watch the speed, watch the different topics. Notice each thought and then release it to make room for the next thought and so on. Repeat this and repeat this and repeat this. Be amused and fascinated with your thoughts at first, then transition naturally into feeling neutral about them.

6. Focus on the feel of your own heart's energy.

7. When you notice you are again thinking, without self-criticism and with kindness, go back to noticing the feel of your heart.

8. Breathe in the following manner: Slowly inhale down into your abdomen. Your abdomen will move outward as you inhale and will ease back into place as you exhale. Exhale for a longer period of time than you inhale. Focus on exhaling and let it last a long time. Exhale slowly and really feel it stretching out a little longer than the inhalation. When you inhale fully, there is a slight pause. Then when you exhale completely, there is a slight pause. Within one cycle of each breath there are two pauses. Feel the natural pause within your breath—the stillness is there inside of your breath.

Remember, only meditate for three to five minutes in the beginning. Allow the length of time to extend on its own. Practice meditating for short moments throughout your day. Feel your soul; it feels different from your mind.

Describe your impressions in your journal after each three-minute meditation.

**Accessing the Imagination Wave**

Now let's deliberately access the energy wave and flow with our imagination. Concentration will never increase your intuitive abilities because concentration is a forced focus of thought from the left hemisphere. When you put aside your own personal thoughts and place yourself in a daydream state of mind, you are naturally accessing the field of collective intelligence that has been building for eternity.

Here are some intuitive guidelines to be aware of:

- Do not assess your imagination with your thoughts.
- Do not censor it with your thoughts.
- Do not evaluate it as true or false with your thoughts.
- Do not interpret the information with your thoughts.
- Do not minimize the intuitive information with your thoughts.
- Do not judge or criticize the information.
- Do not judge or criticize yourself with your thoughts.

I have been a certified clinical hypnotherapist for nearly thirty years. I was literally entranced and fascinated with hypnosis, so I decided to learn what it was all about and how to do it. I discovered that all hypnosis is self-hypnosis. It's true. You do not lose control with a hypnotherapist because they are not taking control of you in the first place. The experience of hypnosis is up to you. You can block it or you can participate with the clinician. You have choice and you have control.

When you participate in hypnosis, you are allowing yourself to enter into the imagination wave. You are sending yourself, with guidance, into an altered state of mind which creates a different electrical signal in your brain. If you were connected to an EEG in a doctor's office, you would see a different electrical pattern beginning to develop.

**Essential Point:**
*Stop thinking you are failing because
it feels like imagination.*

It is the exact same state of mind as your daydreams. Humans naturally enter into a daydream frequency every 1½ to 2 hours during the waking day. Many people call it zoning out, fogging out, or drifting away.

This is the important part:

- The hypnotic state of mind is absolutely natural.

- Daydreams are absolutely natural.

- The imagination wave is absolutely natural.

Your intuitive abilities will constantly feel like your imagination. In truth, it is intuitive information that naturally flows though the electrical frequency that only *feels* like your imagination.

Read through the following steps, then participate with the steps and deliberately practice sending yourself into a daydreamlike, hypnotic imagination space. The following steps will assist you in accessing the imagination wave.

Do not move on to the next step in this course until you are able to intentionally direct your mind into this awareness.

## Steps to the Imagination Wave

1. First notice and understand the sensation of mental toiling. Sit there and force your thoughts and remember how it feels to concentrate on something. When you are aware of how it feels to force thought and the feel of trying too hard, then let go of all the work and effort.

2. Feel yourself being in charge of you. Take charge of your own head and your own thought processes as you make yourself release effort.

3. Remember a time when you felt the sensations of day-dreaming—the spacey, light, uplifting impression. Remember the feelings of a daydream. Remember where your daydreams often take you. Relive a daydream now.

4. Go deeper into that state of being. Deliberately send your awareness into all the sensations of daydreaming. Your body knows the sensory feel of it. Your head knows the feel of it and your mind knows the distinctive nature of it all.

5. Notice images flashing in and out while some images remain.

6. Notice with all of your five senses and even more.

7. Allow the daydream to flow wherever it takes you.

8. Allow and notice. Allow and notice everything.

9. Be aware of your own individual response. There is no way to do this incorrectly.

10. Notice everything, imagine everything.

Document your impressions in your journal now.

Accessing this imagination wave is essential to your personal success as a medical intuitive. Get out of your own way and let the dreamy flow of imagination gush through your being. Stop thinking that you are failing because it feels like imagining. You are experiencing the energy of the non-physical. Stop trying to make it physical when its very nature is non-physical. Intuition is information that ripples or swells in currents of electrical waves. Sometimes it pops, sometimes it darts, and sometimes it even explodes into our perception. Allow your daydream state of mind to unlock your brain and create a state of receptivity to the collective world of information. No one can do this for you.

## Intent: An Action, Not Just a Noun

Now that you have given yourself time to consciously create and send yourself into your meditative, daydreamlike, intuitive realm, you can now consciously direct your dreamy spirit mind to receive the broader scope of information that is available to humans.

In the metaphysical paranormal world, intent has become an empty word and not an action. You keep hearing the directives to "Set your intent to do this . . ." and "Set your intent and you will . . ." No one has ever told me what intent is, or how to actually do it or put it into action. I have never heard anyone even say that intent is an action. To me, intent is deliberately creating focused thought to accomplish something.

Our thoughts are often flying all over the place. A random thought happens here and then a random thought happens there. One minute we are considering the healing situation we are in, and the next moment we are thinking of going to the grocery and the next moment dinner and the next moment what is on TV tonight and if you should make popcorn.

Even when you are trying to focus it seems that your brain has a life of its own—which is true unless you take charge of it. You can take control of your thoughts, and as a result you are taking control of your energy.

Think of the power of lightning. Now consider that each and every thought in your head is a bolt of lightning. Each thought has a slightly different topic and sometimes a completely different topic than the last thought. Each thought has a different electrical bolt with different frequencies, currents, and rhythms. You can allow that energy to work for you and you can stop it from working against you. This is *key*, not only for medical intuition but for life. Get in charge of your thoughts and you get in charge of your energy and you get in charge of your life. You are the creator.

Consciously directing your personal thought energy is what is known as intent. Instead of overflowing with random hectic energy, we can deliberately take charge of it. When we control our thought processes, we create focused, uninterrupted energy with mechanical abilities that scientists have not yet been able to measure or harness.

**Essential Point:**
*Intent is harnessing and directing your thought energy.*

You might say that this is all interesting, but how does it apply to becoming a medical intuitive? A medical intuitive harnesses thought and directs the vibrational intent to connect with another person to receive medical and emotional information for their well-being. Your intent is to receive the entire story that is beneath an illness that has already manifested or a potential illness of body or mind.

Your intent is to emit and purposely project your energetic sensors outward toward the person you are assessing. Your energetic sensors are not only thought energy but also "energy feelers" searching for a myriad of information. Some of the information may include a person's thoughts, emotions, experiences, traumas, heartbreak, and past experiences with the illness or disease.

It is vital that you gain control not only over the projection of your thoughts, but also the intensity and the quality of your thoughts. If you are heading to the grocery store in your head or considering the fight you had with your lover this morning, you are going to fail as a medical intuitive. You will fail yourself and you are going to fail your client. How and where you direct your intent is where your psychic laser-like sensor goes.

Below are the steps for creating intent. As you practice the steps, remember these guidelines: When you become the boss, your thoughts will comply. Enhance the clarity and quality of your thoughts by consistently targeting the positive—appreciation, gratitude, love, and happiness all have the quality and distinct frequency that will enhance your intuitive ability. The positive range of thought energy holds you in a high vibrational status that does not get bogged down. Living at this positive energetic level is like seeing the world from the viewpoint of an eagle; the eagle might have a better, more encompassing view. Intent is an action.

**Steps to Create Intent**

1. Notice your thoughts zooming all over the place and just let them zoom.

2. While your thoughts are rushing around, use it as a time to explore. What is my true plan and purpose and what do I want to accomplish in this particular moment?

3. Specifically select a particular thing among all the random thoughts that you want to focus your intent toward.

4. Notice that your mind wants to stay in charge so it begins to wing around even more now that you have made your selection of intent.

5. Notice without judgment. Judgment sends your thoughts flinging into wildness. The mind loves judgment because it is regaining control again.

6. Like a gentle parent, bring your thoughts back to your intent over and over again.

7. Focus on the feeling of clarity and the feeling of the quality of your focused thought.

8. Notice the feeling of settling in on your intent.

9. Do not push or try hard to do this. It is all about noticing and not toiling. Feel the difference?

10. Get a sense of locking onto the idea that is now your intent.

11. Imagine feeling or seeing the energy of your thought form into a laser beam. Notice the feel of the focus rather than the thought of it.

12. Feel and imagine your focused energy forming into a beam of energy.

13. Feel and imagine that beam of focus rocketing out of your entire body toward your goal.

14. Hold the direction of your thoughts by gently repeating the topic of your focus.

15. Feel the effortlessness on your part, as if you are a docile, neutral bystander simply noticing everything.

16. When you have completed your beam of focus, relax and create a pulling sensation to draw your energy back into your body.

From this point forward, practice creating positive intent each and every day.

Describe your impressions in your journal now.

Before you move on to the next experience, please take at least a week to put these steps into action. It is all about noticing and bringing back each thought that has strayed, then doing it again with fascination, not labor. This is a profound process of creating, generating, and commanding the incredible capability of your mind. This control will extend beyond medical intuition and flow into all aspects of your life. Entering at will into your spirit mind and generating a pure intent is a fundamental skill that you need to master. When you are mastering intent you are mastering your life.

**Enrich Your Light Body**

As I merrily wrote the specific steps to enrich your light body found later in this section, I also did the steps and participated with the process. My computer instantly went wild! The cursor disappeared and the screen spontaneously bolted twenty or more pages ahead. Then it put on the brakes and flew back to the beginning. The curser reappeared but created a little symbol that I have never seen before, and the pages flew by again and landed on the last written page. I felt a surge of energy exchanging between my hands and the touchpad as the pages flung themselves up and down.

I quickly pushed myself away from the computer until we both calmed down. Since my computer did not blow up and my book did not evaporate, I began to giggle. Then I got up, found my flash drive, and backed up the 117 pages that I had already written. Whew!

Similar things have happened at my medical intuition workshops. Can you imagine what might happen when a large group of people are enriching their light bodies? We have blown out entire electrical systems and electrical circuit breakers for entire buildings! We have blown out air conditioners too!

The first day of one workshop, I apologized to the landlady as she called the electrician for help after I led the class through a technique. The next day of the class I decided we should review the procedure and walked the group through it the second day. The lights and air conditioner went out a second time and the landlady, who was still smiling, called for help once again as we all sat giggling in the dark.

My friend and I took a road trip together. On the way, we discussed energy and how the human body is electromagnetic. I went through similar steps that I described at the workshop mentioned above but added some steps about magnetizing positive experiences and positive people to us.

I blew out the CD player in my friend's car at the exact moment I felt a surge of energy coming into my body! We could not get it to work for the remainder of the day. I felt terrible because I knew I damaged it. The next morning, however, all was well again with the CD player. To test what I suspected, I asked my friend if I could repeat the magnetization process. She adamantly denied my request. We both drove in silence, realizing the power that humans really have.

Enriching your light body is real. You can see it and you can feel it happening. The emotion of this great natural lightness is love. It is a simple word and an overused word, but it is all we have in the English language. Love without a single string attached is an intense, fine, and dazzling electrical frequency that quivers through our body in the most vivid spectrum of light. The joy that comes from this level of love is our divine right as human beings. It is up to us to feel it, experience it, and live it.

Yes, each person is light. Each person is an energy being whether we are consciously or unconsciously living in that manner. We are energy, first and foremost, no matter our lifestyle or choices. It is our destiny to mature, enhance our happiness, and flourish. If we attend to this process our light body matures and grows as well. As we live life, we have the choice to become impenetrable with density or to become a sea of refined, shimmering vibration that creates and captivates the juiciest morsels of life. Which is it for you?

Yes, we have many, many choices in life's journey. The medical intuitive needs to enrich and maintain a fine energetic vibration to more accurately perceive the vibrational story beneath the disease of the people we are assisting. We can learn to see into the depths of someone's pain, struggles, and illness. Anyone can utilize the process. It will heighten intuitive awareness for beginners and for professional intuitives and mediums. Enriching the light body will boost the field for any type of energy practitioner as they prepare for a healing session.

*Love* is one of the primary words in the English language that we use in an attempt to define the brilliance of the light. Unconditional love is tough to achieve and to live by.

*Love* without first looking around for approval.

*Love* without insisting that someone change.

*Love* without rules.

*Love* without restraints or censorship.

*Love* without strings attached.

*Love* without criticism or judgement.

*Love* without first thinking about it.

To experience *love* at this level, to give it to ourselves without hesitation and to offer it to another without hesitation, is the soul's aspiration. To experience the divine is to experience the light of love while dwelling in a human body.

### Essential Point:
*To experience the divine is to experience the light of love while dwelling in a human body.*

The goal of enrichment is to enhance and expand your glowing light body. It is vital to feel the glow as you also visualize it. Creating physical sensations within the body always empowers the process. The physical body will create sensations for you, so simply notice these sensations. The more you practice this experience, as detailed below, the easier it becomes. Soon this process will only take a minute or so and will become more powerful each time. Read through the entire process then return to the first step, read it, then do it. Then read the next step and put it into action and so on.

**Steps to Enrich Your Light Body**

1. Begin by really feeling your breath in its normal rhythm. Do not alter the breath's rhythm, only feel it happening.

2. Notice the feeling of your heart and its energy within your chest. As you feel your heart's energy, also imagine seeing your own light in your chest. We are a spark of Source, so imagine the feel of source energy in the very center of your heart and visualize that spark of light within you. Do not work hard at this. Be your own neutral observer simply noticing the energy and light of your heart in its own way.

3. Watch and feel the light intensifying and expanding without any effort—only observe. Feel your breath moving with the light.

4. Your breath and the light will begin to grow larger moving past the heart center, filling every inch of your physical body. Allow your body to take the lead and take as long as your body wants as it fills with the light.

5. Purposely direct the light and send it all along your back as well. When you *feel* full of breath and light, go on to the next step.

6. Notice that your breath and light expands naturally beyond your skin, twinkling outward in every direction around you. Feel it and visualize it behind you, beside you, beneath you, and above you.

7. True grounding is a complete cycle of connecting to the earth and allowing the earth to connect with you. Allow your body to continue to breathe normally. As you exhale, feel your breath and your light pouring down both legs equally and traveling deep inside the earth. Continue exhaling until you feel energy flowing downward easily. You are literally exhaling down your legs and out through the soles of your feet, going ever so deep into the earth. Continue until you have a sense of connection to the globe that you live on.

8. Now shift your awareness to inhaling. Notice your inhalation and draw your breath upward and through the soles of your feet and back up your legs each time that you inhale. Let the energy begin to fill you naturally and without any force. Let it move on its own accord. No pushing. Actively draw up the earth energy into your body by actually inhaling and feeling your breath coming up through the soles of your feet. Feel energy flowing higher and higher into your entire body until you have a sense of fullness.

9. Exhale back down into the earth through the soles of your feet, then draw the earth back up through your legs. Feel the entire circuit and cycle of the breath. Feel energy and

the light. The roots of trees grow down into the ground, but those same roots absorb all that the earth has to offer, drawing that life energy into the full length of the tree. Thus a complete exchange happens and a complete cycle forms.

10. Now do the same through the top of your head. Directing the energy with your breath, exhale out from the top of your head and then inhale the light of the Universe in through your crown, letting it travel deep into your heart center. Do not work at it; continue to only feel and see light coming in through the top of your head when inhaling and the exchange of energy as you exhale the light back into the universe.

11. Sense that you are a lightning rod and antennae for electromagnetic cosmic energy surging back and forth through your body and mind. The energy of the earth and the energy of the Universe intermingles within your body.

12. Now the glow streams in and out of every inch of your skin. Every inch of your skin radiates the glow, accepting it and also sending it out. The center of your physical heart shines out from your being and absorbs it back from the universe. The frequency of love from your heart is the hub of your glow. See it and feel it brighter than the sun.

13. Allow yourself to feel and know your entire body as a fine wire, a fine filament for current to ebb and flow like the ocean's tide. Allow and notice currents and waves of well-being tingle through your body. You are the link between the heavens and the earth.

Describe your impressions in your journal now.

# Chapter Five

## Prepare to Get in Charge of You

### Take Charge of Your Energy Field

How many times do you hear people say, "I just don't know why I did that" or "Why did I say that?" People usually have no idea why they are the way they are or why they say what they say. There is even less awareness about taking charge of who they are and what they do. We are responsible for our lives, our thoughts, and our bodies. Let's take that responsibility back and let's assist others to understand that they can also be in charge of themselves.

People often tell me that they cannot help doing something because that is just who they are. Do you hear the passivity in that statement? People are implying that life is haphazard and happens by chance. Many do not understand that we have the power to deliberately change our patterns, change our thinking, and change our beliefs. We do not need to be victims of our thoughts. Life can have a richer quality when we step up to the plate and own our body, our thoughts, and the soul presence that dwells within us.

We also have the ability to take charge of our energy field. In fact, medical intuition is about taking charge of energy. When we receive a medical intuition reading we learn how our energy field is functioning and not functioning. We hear what it looks like and how it is expanding or contracting. We learn where density is accumulating and the story behind the struggle. The client receives an unbiased viewpoint from the medical intuitive. When we begin to understand our struggles from a different perspective, we can begin to change our thought patterns, which in turn begin to alter our energy.

The medical intuitive practitioner takes charge of their own energy field to perform the scan. In general, the practitioner builds up the level of energy within their body and projects it outward toward the receiver. The intuitive collects an uncountable amount of evidence that floats in and around each person's aura and relays that information back to them.

The medical intuitive practitioner does not take on the energy of the person they are scanning. It is a matter of receiving their energetic information without integrating the client's energy into your own energy. When a session is actually completed, you may discover an inability to remember the details because you immediately released their energy and moved back into your own life.

Energy is not limited by distance. The receiver of the scan can be two feet away or on the other side of the globe. The distance does not matter. We are only limited by our limited thoughts. If you think that you cannot do an intuitive scan over a distance, then you will not be able to do distance work. When you change your restricted thinking to expansive thinking, you expand your abilities. Expanded thought equals expanded energy equals expanded experiences.

Energy not only follows thought but also follows imagination. As you sense the energy in your chest spreading throughout the body, one can then imagine energy emanating out past the skin. Your energy will follow your imagination. This is an absolute key to psychic perceptions. As you imagine your energy projecting outward, upward, downward, or across the oceans of the earth, your energy immediately responds to the expansion of imagination.

**Essential Point:**
*Medical intuitives receive energetic information without integrating the client's energy into their own energy field.*

As you purposely direct your energy field, an immediate response happens. It will seem as if you are extending delicate sensors from the edge of your energy field. As you imagine your field extending in different directions, you will soon realize the control you have with it. You are developing a partnership of mind, imagination, and electrical energy, all working together to perceive the unseen world and to assist others with medical intuition. As you play with your field you are becoming the director of your deepest, most natural intuitive abilities.

**Essential Point:**
*Purposely directing energy will feel as if you have sensors at the edge of your field.*

Let's play with directing your energy now. Read through the following steps first, then playfully apply the steps.

**Playful Steps to Direct Your Energy**

1. Remind yourself that you cannot do this incorrectly. Feel playful with the following steps.

2. Sit comfortably, breath normally, and notice any sensations of warmth, aliveness, or energy in your chest. Feel the energy in your heart and chest and how it seems to actually take up space in your chest, filling it from front to back.

3. Using your imagination, send your breath down and all around the organ of your heart, building up the glow of vitality. Remember to imagine.

4. Now expand the energy up, down, and all around within your body. Fill your arms, hands, fingertips, ears, hips, toes, knees—everywhere. Remember to fill your entire backside with energy too.

5. Saturate your entire body until it can no longer be contained beneath the skin. Feel it radiating outward past the skin.

6. Playfully push the energy two to three inches beyond your skin. Sense it following your intent.

7. Now imagine your energy stretching outward like taffy or

a rubber band. Send it outward to approximately three feet past your skin. Feel the bigness of your energy field.

8.  Expand and stretch your energy toward the corner of the room and notice everything that comes into your awareness from that viewpoint. It will seem as if you are in the body and in the corner of the room at the same time.

9.  Remember to feel in charge of you and be the director of your thoughts and your energy.

10. Gently and playfully send the edge of your energy into the wall of the room that you are in. You are the director of your energy. Imagine being inside of the wall. Feel the textures; see the materials the wall is made of; smell the materials within the wall; sense it in absolutely your own way.

11. Draw the edge of your energy back to you and rest a while, full of awareness.

12. Now direct your energy field upward to the ceiling and hover there for a moment. Look around the room from that level of the ceiling.

13. Gently push your field through the ceiling, noticing everything about it as you do so.

14. Next, send yourself on through the roof in the same manner. Sit on the roof. Feel it on your buttocks. Notice the weather of the day and look around. Notice everything from that vantage point.

15. Stay on the roof and notice. Be deliberate, precise, and aware. Be in control of what you do and where you go. Do not fly all over the place or go to a different area.

16. When you feel successful on the roof, begin to gently pull your energy back into your body, making sure that you draw it all completely back into your physical body. You will feel complete when you do so.

Describe your impressions in your journal now.

Repeat the process described above until you feel the joy and freedom of this expanded experience. At first you might find yourself zooming all over the place instead of sitting on the roof. When I first realized this human ability, I went everywhere and I went fast. I was a happy, happy traveler. That is fine at first, but the goal of this process is to develop deliberate control of your field.

## Laser Beam: The Ultimate Key for Excellence

The accurate medical intuitive needs to develop control in multiple areas. Focused thinking creates powerful intent. Intent with imagination creates expansion. Playful expansion creates the ability to overcome any distance between you and the person you are assessing. The intuitive must be able to direct their energy in a systematic manner toward the recipient in order to excel as a medical intuitive. I call this directed, focus energy the laser beam technique.

When I first began to teach my laser beam technique I did not help people connect this concept to becoming a medical intuitive. I guess most people thought I was simply teaching a fun thing they could do with their energy field. I was shocked when I began to realize that people did not understand this as a key step toward doing a medical intuition session. I did not help them connect to the fact that this ability is one of the most important steps in receiving very accurate and detailed medical/emotional information for your client. So I want to emphasize this detail now: Your laser beam, with hypersensitive receptive sensors, picks up details such as mineral/vitamin deficiencies, ulcers, tumors, emotions, broken hearts, broken bones, clogged blood vessels, dysfunctional heart valves, dehydration, and the list goes on and on.

In the near future you will be using your own laser beam of focus to reach out to a client or friend in need. You will use this ability not only to reach out but to enter into their auric energy body for information about their struggles. You will then go past the skin into their physical body for a truly in-depth scan of tissues, organs, chakras, bones, and blood. You already had this ability, but now you are aware of this ability. I insist that you use this level of awareness with honor, integrity, and confidentiality, for there is nothing more intimate than a medical intuitive session together.

It is important for you to realize on the deepest level to not continue this training until you can cast your energy with clear intent, clear focus, and clear control. Before moving on, you must know and feel that you are truly sitting on the roof, noticing the view or projecting outward to the corner of a room and then be able to pull your energy back into your body. Make sure you have brought all of you back to you. Take your time to practice until you know you are the creator of your highly sensitive intuitive skills. Take your time to practice, practice, practice.

**Recognize Your Mind's Eye**

The following exercise will assist you in recognizing the abilities of your mind's eye. Repeat this process with different objects until you easily recognize your innate ability to perceive this way.

1.  Choose one object that is near you at this moment. It could be a vase, a lamp, or absolutely any inanimate object sitting nearby.

2.  Memorize the object until you know all of its details.

3.  Now close your eyes and imagine that same object in your head.

4.  Open your eyes again and stare at the object.

5.  Close your eyes and notice that the mind mechanically imprints the image of the object in your mind.

6.  Do not put forth any type of effort as you do this exercise. Remain passive as you look at the object and then remain passive as you see the image of the object within your mind.

7. Repeat this process with different objects in your environment.

Document your impressions in your journal now.

Do not move on until you truly experience the imprint of each object in your head. Remember to practice this experience playfully. Working hard at it will only interfere and decrease visual awareness. When you have completed this exercise, continue to the next mind's eye experience.

Now expand the awareness of your mind's eye with this next process: Imagine a tree out in a field. Notice I am not asking you to look outdoors at a physical tree. I am asking you to imagine the image of a tree within your mind's eye.

Document your impressions about the tree in your journal now.

In my medical intuitive workshop, most students happily report, "Yes, I see a tree." But they do not report any details about the tree they see within their minds. They do not see their tree in any descriptive manner. When questioned, however, they offer all types of facts about their tree.

First notice, without judgment, how scant or how detailed your written description is. Below is a list of questions about the tree. As you read each question, jot down the knowing that comes to you about the tree.

- Describe the size of the tree.

- How old is the tree?

- What do the leaves look like?

- What color are the leaves?

- Are the leaves mature as in late summer or new and small as if in spring or brightly colored as if in the fall?

- What season does your tree present itself in?

- How far or near are you from the tree?

- What does the bark feel like to your touch?

- Is the tree in full leaf or are some of the branches bare?
- What does the field look like? Is the field flat, rolling, or even mountainous?
- Any fences appearing?
- What is growing in the field all around the tree, if anything?
- What colors does the growth appear in?
- Are there any buildings or people near the tree?

When you have completed the list presented above, notice the following: First, be aware of how many details you did not notice about the tree when you first visualized it. Second, notice that as you read these questions, you simply knew more about your tree. Third, your description of the tree immediately became more defined and you had more information.

Here are four vital points emphasized in the practice above:

1. This all feels like your imagination and yet it feels very real for you.

2. Your tree might look and feel the opposite of mine and yet it is right for you and you alone.

3. You may not have noticed important distinctive details without my detailed questions.

4. Profound intuitive information is found in the details of your perceptions.

You experienced an object in your imagination. Then your tree within your mind became very unique to you and might have been very different from mine. While you might have witnessed a giant oak, mine might have been a young willow blowing in a breeze. Yours was deeply correct for you just as my willow was correct for me. You then proceeded to become aware of minute facets and different elements that composed the more complete story of the tree. In other words, the entire story of the tree as it stands now became known to you.

There is yet more information that your tree can give to you. Look over all of your documentation about the tree. Read and assimilate all of the details that popped into your mind's eye. Jot down the most immediate answer to this question:

*What does my tree, in all of its detail, tell me about my story?*

Each one of us experiences diverse perceptions, and each perception is valuable for our individual reality. Those unique, detailed perceptions will also be important as you work with medical intuition. Your accuracy as a medical intuitive is in the details of the intuitive information that you receive.

**Essential Point:**
*Intuitive excellence is in the details of what you perceive.*

If you overlook the details that lie deep within your intuition, you will miss the mark in receiving critical information as a medical intuitive. If you fail to notice the amazing detail regarding the image of the tree in your mind's eye, you will continue to minimize crucial evidence as a medical intuitive. No piece of information stands alone. Your tree stands within an environment. Not only does the tree offer many details, but so does the entire setting around the tree.

The setting, the distance, the season, etc., provide even more intuitive details about the story. Each and every detail delivers information for the intuitive. Nothing can be ignored or minimized. When you ignore the details, you ignore specific information. The detail transforms your medical scan from mediocre to superior for the client.

**Essential Point:**
*Your brain naturally and mechanically perceives in images.*

Be conscious of how you simply knew the answers to such questions as "What season does your tree present itself in?" Many will instantly see the tree again and receive the response visually. Others might feel a knowing wave wash through them or the answers will spring into the mind. Allow yourself to receive the details and when you do, you are one more step toward receiving and giving a quality reading for the benefit of others.

**Essential Point:**
*Your personal self-awareness will accentuate your medical intuitive awareness for others.*

There is one more critical observation to consider. Where did your mind's eye seem to appear or form within you or around you? Identify the location where the above perceptions presented themselves. Localize a place where the tree seemed to be displayed in your mind's eye. You may notice that as you stared at and memorized an object in your living space and then as you noted the details regarding your tree, both images seemed to visually appear in the same place in your mind's eye.

Four sites are reported as the most common location of the mind's eye:

1. Behind the eyelids.

2. In the center of the brain.

3. Behind the forehead.

4. Floating in the air in front of the head.

There is no right or wrong way and there is no right or wrong location for these perceptions. It is all about awareness of you as an individual, first and foremost. Your self-awareness will accentuate your medical intuitive awareness for others.

Describe your impressions in your journal now.

Hopefully you have discovered yourself in slightly different ways. You have studied an actual object sitting around your home and practiced visualizing the imprint created in your mind's eye. You then visualized a tree and noticed the detailed story about the tree. You then had an opportunity to learn where the visual perception of your mind's eye is located and how it tends to materialize. Your mind's eye might even be located in a different place than listed above.

In this chapter you have learned about allowing the imagination wave, how intent is an energetic action, how you are naturally wired for visualization, receiving a more complete intuitive story about your visualizations, and noticing how and where visualizations manifest for you as an individual. These steps are important preparation to receiving medical intuition.

## You Are Not Failing

Time and time again a few students declare, "Nothing happened! I didn't notice a thing in my mind's eye, only blackness." Others in the class then declare, "I just saw the bones of the person sitting next to me, and I really saw it like an x-ray!" I ask the people who feel they are failing to describe what they did notice. The people in failure always respond that they only have thoughts in their heads and do not have any images. I then say, "Well, tell me about the thoughts and what you noticed as the thoughts came in."

These same people then begin to express all the intuitive information they picked up. One person "in failure" carefully explained they only picked up a light haze of purple around the right side of their subject's head for a fleeting moment, and it was completely transparent so they know they did not get anything. Another person mentioned that a phrase kept repeating in their mind and it became an annoyance that distracted them and so they stopped trying.

When I asked what the phrase was, he responded, "Oh, it was only the words of a song that goes like this: 'Walk in my shoes . . .'" Then another person who also declared failure jumped in to report, "Well, I only saw a dark spot around my person's heart and then a dog seemed to be sitting next to us, so I certainly didn't get a thing!"

**Essential Point:**
*Your preconceived expectations completely block your success.*

You, the reader, as a neutral outsider looking into this situation, might immediately understand that the "people of failure" received a wealth of information!

It is imperative to know that we all discount intuitive information. You must know how you as an individual tend to discredit your intuition. In the above examples, people ignored their intuitive hits when the hits didn't follow their expectations. The intuition was not what they wanted, not "solid" enough, not where they thought it would happen, not how they thought it should take place, not enough of something, or not how it should look.

Instead of yes to everything that popped in, it was no, no, no, no.

During this same class, I asked the people who were receiving the scan to comment. One woman announced that she was delighted to hear that the right side of her head was glowing in purple because she had just gone back to painting class and felt her creativity had skyrocketed. (The right side of the brain is conceptual thinking and purple signifies imagination and creativity. The transparency denotes that it is new and has not developed density.) While the person who picked up this information discounted all of it, the receiver stated that all of the information made sense to her.

I then asked about the song phrase "Walk in my shoes." The receiver told her classmate that she'd worn new shoes to the class that day and they had rubbed blisters all over her feet! Then the woman with the dark spot over her heart and the dog sitting near her suddenly burst into tears as she tried to explain that her dog of fifteen years had died the previous week and that she was deeply grieving. I ask you, did the people who decided they failed really fail? Absolutely not. They did, however, fail to:

- Notice
- Allow
- Receive whatever came in
- Accept that intuition comes in unexpected forms
- Trust everything that pops in
- Honor what they receive

Each student received detailed, medically based, intuitive information for the person they were working with. Each student was amazed and agreed that they unexpectedly visualized medical information but did not consciously acknowledge it even as it happened. Prior to this moment each of them were adamantly denying they ever visualized anything. If you insist that you cannot intuitively see, *stop* thinking it now. You are wired to receive psychic information. Accept everything in a different manner and stop expecting it to happen in certain ways. Your preconceived expectations completely block your success.

**Scan Yourself First Before Others**

Do you find that you want to skip this section? Don't do it! It is vital for your evolvement as a medical intuitive.

Please do not skip this experience claiming that it is unnecessary or a waste of time. Notice all the reasons that your mind comes up with to avoid doing this part. Notice this avoidance without judgment or criticism. The more we truly know about ourselves, the clearer we can be for others. Sometimes this self-assessment is actually the scariest.

Knowing your own truth, your tendencies, and your own struggles will clarify your ability as a medical intuitive. You must be able to distinguish what symptoms are yours and what belongs to another. Many medical intuitives pick up information about their clients by receiving physical sensations within their own body. You must know what your own aches and pains and booboos are first. Any changes during the medical intuitive session are signals about your client and not you.

Now that we have discussed the spirit mind and intent, let's look deep within our own body and energy. Make a copy of the human form that is offered on the next page for this experience. Have pen and colored markers in front of you before you begin. Read through the easy steps first to get the complete feeling of what you are about to do. This experience might feel as if you are walking around inside of your own body. Remember to notice everything as a neutral observer but also be fascinated with your findings!

Begin at the top of your head and move throughout your entire body. You might have a tendency to scan only along your skin, so make sure you go beyond the skin and enter deep inside of your body. Focus within each internal area of your body. As you proceed through each section of your body, be aware of the perceptions that jump into your mind as if out of nowhere. Accept the most instant perception within each bodily section. Do not give your mind any time to alter the information. Write or color whatever jumps into your awareness.

Here is a general summary of what to look for. A more specific step-by-step guide comes after.

1. Be prepared to jot down or color in whatever information you receive on the human body form. Quickly move throughout your body.

2. First notice a color even if it feels as if you are pretending to see a color.

3. Notice the most immediate word, phrase, or story that jumps into your awareness and write it down.

4. Does a symbol appear? Draw it immediately.

5. If there seems to be a struggle, how does that struggle present itself?

6. Ask each area what it needs or wants. Your body will talk to you. Simply listen and look.

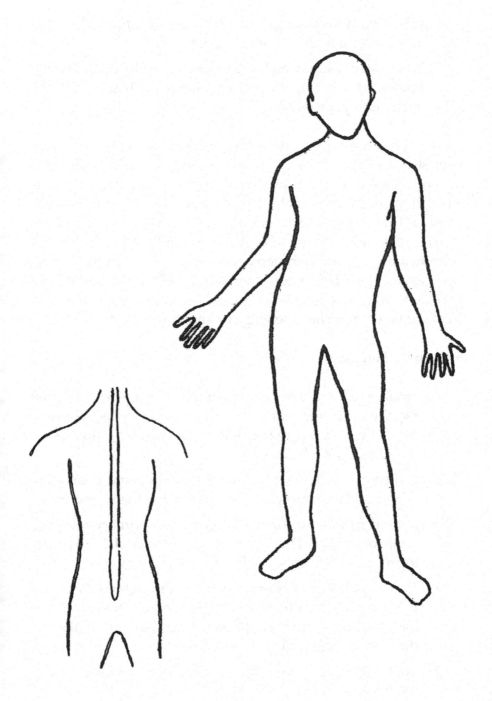

7. Create your own question for what you want to know about a certain section of your body.

8. If you are not sure which organ you are evaluating, simply ask your body telepathically and accept the first word that enters into your mind.

If you still want to skip the self-scan, take a moment to evaluate your struggle about it. What is coming up that might be difficult for you to look at? What do you want to avoid? What are you worried about or afraid of? Do this for yourself because you are worth it! Do it for yourself many, many times before moving on.

The following are the specific self-scanning steps to assess your own body. Read each step one at a time and do what it asks. Once again, document your insights on the human body form provided. Your documentation might include colors, feelings, words, images, movement, energy, or knowing.

**Steps for a Self-Scan**

1. Notice your entire body from your head to the soles of your feet. You are more than just a thinking head. Feel yourself as a "unit of being" that includes your feet, legs, hips, torso, arms, and also a head.

2. Write your most instant general thought about your "unit of being." What impressions pop in? Write them down now.

3. Imagine a main color that seems to be primary for your "unit of being." Draw that color all around the human form.

4. Now look inside of your head, going throughout the brain. Look at one hemisphere and then the other. Does each side look similar or are they different? Do they feel similar or different? Draw what you notice.

5. Look into your sinuses, face, mouth, eyes, and ears. Draw whatever pops in.

6.  Roam around within your neck and throat. Compare the right side with the left. Then enter the thyroid gland at the base of the neck.

7.  Scan down inside of your arms and into your hands. Note your observations.

8.  Go back to your chest area and upper back, taking in the muscles. Go inside your lungs before the heart. Is each lung equal in appearance in all ways?

9.  Now enter into your heart area.

10. Proceed to the stomach next, in the location of the solar plexus above the belly button.

11. Shift to the gallbladder and liver on the right side of the abdomen.

12. Now evaluate the spleen and pancreas on the left side of the abdomen.

13. Check out the intestines that lie throughout the lower abdomen then go down into the colon, which sits in the left lower quadrant of the abdomen.

14. Check out the bladder, which rests in the center of the pelvic area just above the genital area.

15. Next go to the male or female reproductive organs (whichever applies) and review them.

16. Notice the muscles all around the trunk of your body and then look into the hip area.

17. Go down inside of each leg individually, all the way to your toes and soles of your feet.

18. Now look around inside of your bones, including your spine.

19. Review your blood system.

20. Now the lymph system.

21. You can also check out the seven primary chakra centers

located at base of the spine or groin, below the belly button, above the belly button, the heart, the throat, the third eye in the center of the forehead, and then the top of your head, known as the crown.

You have intimately perceived your own private vehicle that you inhabit. Please be open to repeating the self-scan process multiple times throughout the remainder of this course. Each time you repeat this private process, you will grow in awareness. You will truly understand what each ache or pain is telling you about you. You will grow into a more intimate understanding of what makes you tick, why you say what you say and do what you do.

Just before I see a client I do an instant scan of myself so I know my current status. I check my body and my emotions to have a baseline so that I can recognize that any changes during our session are intuitive messages about my client's health.

# Chapter Six

## Prepare for Spirit Assistance

### You Are Not Alone: Invite Your Specialist

We humans are hard workers and it usually does not occur to us to ask for help. Notice how you might already be working hard to read this book, trying to study it, memorizing certain statements, and possibly struggling through the exercises. Stop toiling this very moment. Be in charge of your own head and thinking mind. It is no wonder we feel exasperated and annoyed with ourselves. Now turn your efforts over to Spirit. Turn your struggles over to the collective infinite intelligence. Turn it over to all that has been achieved and valued, the immeasurable heart essence of the collective consciousness.

Remember the biblical phrase "As above, so below"? Just as we have specialists in every imaginable career and endeavor on the earth plane, we also have specialists in the non-physical kingdom. When you began to consider medical intuition, your specialty guide began to stir in the heavens. Maybe your medical intuition guide was already drawn to you and standing beside you, initiating the stirring of your psychic inquisitiveness. Regardless of how your interest began or who began it, here you are, and you are alone only if you choose to be.

Spirit is ready and willing to respond to our requests, but the secret is that we have to ask for it. This is a world of choice and to struggle alone or to ask for divine assistance is one component amid the vast number of daily choices we have. Choice may be a blessing and sometimes it may seem a curse. Choice, when handled with awareness, is a gift in life.

We need to first understand that we have an unfathomable array of constant and continuous choice in every single moment of our day. Second, we must choose with awareness. The more we choose with awareness, the smoother life becomes. That awareness comes to us in the form of instinct, intuition, and experience. To ask for assistance or to go it alone with medical intuition is up to you, though I will say those wanting to improve their perception will eventually need to ask for spirit guides.

**Essential Point:**
*When you began to consider medical intuition, your specialty guide began to stir in the heavens.*

Spirit guides come in many forms and are diversified in talents or focus. Some of your guides will be with you forever, and some come and go depending on your needs and interests. Even if you are already aware of your current guides, please realize that you might also have a medical intuition specialist that you can call on. These spirit specialists have usually dedicated their soul essence to specific areas. For instance, years ago I requested a financial specialty guide to assist me, not only with money but also with learning about the energy of receiving abundance in all areas of my life.

At another time, I specifically called out for a Reiki master guide, asking for one who excels in the vibration of Reiki to oversee the work I was doing for others. He appeared before me and, when asked, gave me a name to identify him in the future. Many months went by with little thought of my specialty guide. When I did think of him, I immediately regretted trying to do Reiki on my own and I would quickly and sheepishly call him in to assist me. I instantly felt the energy swelling up and literally surging through me with a greater force than I could ever do alone.

One day while hiking alone in the northern New Mexico mountains. I stood still and alone, soaking up the wilderness around me. I noticed a ripple of energy flowing through me. The energy of the canyon intensified. The colors around me glowed in neon vibrations. It all became physical sensation. My Reiki specialty guide stood before me and began to move all around me, performing some type of ceremony. It did not appear as an attunement, but the experience felt like a tremendous attunement, altering me for some purpose or reason. When we welcome guidance and direction, our spirit guides delightfully provide surprises, energy, and their wisdom.

There are no limits to the specialists who reside in the non-physical kingdom. When you put out a request with the highest and greatest sensation of love from your mind and heart, that request releases an electromagnetic wave that reverberates across the Universe, instantly drawing a spirit response. Even as you read this, a stirring begins. As the stirring begins, consider the qualities or traits you want assistance with. Focus on qualities rather than stating specifics. For instance, if you specifically invite in a spirit doctor, you might have limited yourself in who responds. That doctor might have specialized in one area and may not excel in all areas of health.

### Essential Point:
*Your energetic invitation creates radio-type signals into the cosmos.*

Invite a guide who excels at the highest level of medical understanding, healing, medical diagnosis, energy work, intuitive vision, or all of the above. Your energetic invitation creates radio-type signals into the cosmos. The signal you create depends on the qualities you have asked for in a guide. The signal also depends on the personal energetic level you have achieved. In other words, if you vibrate in levels of resentment, frustration, or even hatred, you can only draw that which is similar. If you dwell in vibrations of love, compassion, and healing, you will naturally and effortlessly attract spirit guides at that level.

**Essential Point:**
*Listen to Spirit by noticing all thoughts
that dash into your head.*

Realize that as your needs change or alter, your guides may change as well. They do not take offense if you insist the information they are giving you come in faster or clearer. For example, you might ask for more visual information or you might ask for a message to give to the client.

You can even discuss with your guide that you would like to work with someone else. You can ask if there is someone who can offer you even greater assistance or assistance in a different way. Ask for the highest and most loving benefit for you and the people you are assisting with medical intuition. Spirit guides have a more neutral and intellectual understanding of relationships and will not take offense.

Just as important as spirit guidance are our personal responsibilities. We must constantly fine tune our own vibration. Do not automatically blame your spirit guide specialist for failing to give you the information clearly. We must clean up our own body, fine tune our thought energy, and learn to control our emotions. It is up to us to get out of our own way and to focus on being the clearest vessel for sending and receiving non-physical information. It is up to each of us to completely focus on the person we are serving. It is up to us to relinquish control of a reading and to turn it over to the most elevated information possible. Remember, like attracts like. We can only receive the most elevated information when we advance to that same vibrational level.

**Essential Point:**
*We must clean up our own body, fine tune our thought energy,
and learn to control our emotions.*

There are many factors that help us to improve our energy field. These factors include but are not limited to the following:

- Constantly taking charge and directing our thoughts.
- Constantly creating positive thoughts.
- Constantly guiding our emotions to respond rather than react.
- Constantly meditating for brief moments.
- Constantly enriching our light body.
- Constantly realizing we are creators.

As discussed earlier, most people feel they are victims of their own random thoughts. It's as if someone else is at the steering wheel of our heads. It is paramount that we take charge of our thought processes and direct our thoughts in positive directions.

When you work with the general public you will sit in intimacy with individuals from all walks of life, and believe me, after working in the mental health field since 1979, I know that there are as many ways to live and exist as there are people. You will find that people have different values, different levels of integrity, and different ways of interacting with the world.

When you access their story you must do so without judgment and without reacting. You are the neutral observer assisting others toward well-being no matter what they are about, no matter what they think, no matter what they do for a living, and no matter what they feel. When each person requests your assistance, can you participate with them without criticism or judgment?

Read through the following steps first so you have a sense of the process of calling your guide, which will include many of the processes described earlier in this book. It will include enriching your light body, sending yourself into daydreamlike meditative awareness, and creating clear intent.

For now, do not try to visualize your guide. Trying and trying to see your guide will only activate the thinking mind and get in your way. Focus only on sensing, feeling, and imagining your guide. Allow yourself to actually feel successful with this experience. Allow a specialist into your life now. Remember: it will always feel as if you are imagining it.

**Steps to Your Medical Intuitive Specialist**

1. Allow your thoughts to truly understand that there is no way to do this wrong. It is a matter of participating with your new spirit guide specialist.

2. Allow your thoughts to flow as fast as they wish until you sense they are slowing down of their own accord. Remember, never fight against your thoughts for you will not win that fight. Each thought is now considered only a surge of energy.

3. Send yourself, actively participating in your own process, into that daydreamlike meditative place and space.

4. State your request to the spirit realm, asking for the perfect guide to assist you as a medical intuitive.

5. Feel the words as you state them and feel the stirring of energy from the universe around you.

6. Do not try to see your guide. Notice any perceptions that pop into your mind.

7. Notice the impression of a presence coming toward you.

8. From what direction does the guide approach?

9. Notice where the guide stands or hovers. How close is the guide to you?

10. Focus only on sensing the energy of its presence.

11. Detect your own emotions as you sense this divine presence.

12. Notice if the guide feels feminine or masculine or neither gender. Again, do not try hard to visualize. Focus on sensing in other ways first.

13. Notice if the guide moves or remains in the same place and proximity to you.

14. Talk to your specialist by sending telepathic thought energy outward toward the direction that you sense them.

15. Gratitude and appreciation generate the finest levels of energy. Send the physical sensations of those emotions to them.

16. Send a statement or a question to your guide, then relax, feeling very passive, and quietly wait.

17. You are listening now to Spirit. Listen by becoming aware of any and all thoughts that dash into your head. Watch for instantaneous thought. Spiritual guidance often comes in the form of thought energy rushing toward us and popping into our brains. Accept only the initial, instant thoughts. They will be the clearest because the mind does not have time to interfere.

18. Bring your session to a close, sending a deep sense of joy and gratitude to this guide.

Describe your impressions in your journal now.

As you continue the training steps throughout this book, you have the option to struggle on your own or to call in your specialty guides. You can utilize the powerful energy of Spirit even as you continue your training in medical intuition with this book. Invite your specialist to join in and give you clear and direct guidance as you continue through each exercise presented.

The divine is eager to assist us when we ask for it, and it is especially exciting when we allow ourselves to receive from them. Develop a relationship with your specialists. Repeat the above process before each exercise to experience the full dimension of conscious awareness.

## Spirit Specialists Communicate in Many Ways

There are many, many ways in which Spirit attempts to communicate their ethereal information across to us denser (and I say that with a smile) human beings. Spirit works through areas of least resistance. I will repeat that because it is so important. Spirit works through areas of least resistance. The non-physical nature of the spirit realm requires movement and flow. For example, if our thoughts are resistant, Spirit will tend to come to us through our dreams because our thinking mind during sleep is not actively discounting or denying the realm of spirit.

Spirit seems to use particular methods of communication during medical intuition sessions such as telepathy, mental symbols, pictures, body sensations, sounds, smells, and magnetizing focus. Let's look at each of these approaches individually.

### Telepathic Thought

Many definitions of telepathy are stated in *The Encyclopedic Psychic Dictionary* by June Bletzer, PhD. One definition states telepathy is "the coinciding of any of the five psychic senses of two individuals at the exact same time, one is receiving and one is sending; both individuals can be alive or one can be deceased." Another definition stated here is "caused by the transmission of electromagnetic waves between all atoms connecting the universe together (connecting particles, neutrons, bioenergetics vibrations and radiations); these electromagnetic waves and particles, etc., can be tuned into (when one is in a passive frame of mind) by the body or the conscious mind." One more definition: "The touch of consciousness of one person upon another with the ability to discern what that person is thinking or feeling at the present moment."

Remember that intuition is simply the ability to receive information. We are sitting in an enormous bathtub, bathed in a luscious bubble bath of information from the cosmos. I have discussed telepathy earlier in this book, but it is so important I feel the need to discuss it in terms of interacting and developing a relationship with our specialty guides.

Many students feel that they fail to receive intuitive information and subsequently decide that they are intuitive failures. People then drop out of the intuitive world all together. With an explanation and an understanding about spirit communicating with us, each student begins to excel. That makes me smile.

Occasionally telepathic thought does come in a strong voice

that one can hear as if a dear friend is standing next to you speaking loudly in your ear. I must say, however, that an auditory voice from Spirit is a bit rare. When it does happen, it is often an alert that a dangerous situation is about to happen.

**Essential Point:**
*The more you turn your struggles and efforts over to Spirit, the more direction you will receive.*

When you speak within your own mind, each thought radiates out beyond your skull, moving outward and into infinity. Have you considered that each of your thoughts, positive or negative, flows forever and joins all other thoughts ever thought? This is what Carl Jung considered part of the collective consciousness— literally a collection of all thought from the beginning of time.

Let's get back to you communicating with Spirit. When you want to talk to your guide, you need to speak the thoughts only within your mind. It is the same with prayer. While sometimes we pray aloud, most of our prayers are soft words spoken inside our minds. Most people say that they never hear back from God or their spirit guides never respond. If that is the case with you, I have good news for you. It truly only means that you have not been listening.

Listening should be 50 percent of communication. Even in the physical world, listening is often a struggle for people. Listening is even more of a struggle with the non-physical world. The spirit realm is communicating with us constantly. We just do not know how to listen and receive it. When we talk to God or our guides or the soul of another human, we chatter away with our own thoughts and feelings. When we are finished chattering, we go on about our daily business. We have not stopped to listen, which is the other 50 percent of communication. We have not given ourselves time to listen for the response.

There are several aspects to consider when you want to improve your listening. First, talk or ask questions to your specialists, then stop, quiet oneself, and receive. Listening is a general term that really means allowing and noticing thought energy leaping into your mind from another being.

Second, thought energy gushes out of us constantly. To receive thought energy that is gushing back to us, listen to the non-physical world by receiving and accepting thoughts that rush or pop into your mind. It is as simple as that.

Third, accurate listening is the ability to accept the very first thought that pops into your head the instant you become quiet. Speak within your mind, then pause only for an instant. You then receive instant telepathic information. Speak, pause for a split second, receive and accept the first piece of information that rockets into your mind.

Speak, pause, receive, accept.

This pattern will be repeated many times in this training manual. The first, most instant thought that pops into your mind is the clearest information of all. It is the clearest because information did not have time to come from your own thinking mind. Spirit telepathically jolts information into your mind when it is uncluttered by your own thoughts. The clearest, most uncluttered moment is the instant you pause to listen. Your thinking mind has not had time to analyze or judge or ponder.

### Essential Point:
*The clearest, most uncluttered moment is the instant*
*you pause to listen.*

I felt a little lost during one of my medical intuitive sessions. As I scanned throughout the person's body, each component was, at first, quite clear. Suddenly, when I got down to this person's lower abdomen just around the pubic bone, I hesitated. It looked as if his bladder was dark and unhealthy, yet I paused before I stated it. As I looked more closely with x-ray eyes, I felt that something was going on in this area, but the information was not apparent to me.

Instead of floundering, I specifically asked for more clarity from my guide specialist, and instantly the word "tailbone" popped into my head. I focused on the tailbone and a flow of images and information rushed in. I asked for information, waited very passively, and received the information in words and images that surged into my mind.

**Essential Point:**
*Ask for information, then passively wait to receive words or images bursting into the mind.*

It is up to each of us to listen during a conversation. To listen deeply you must quiet your own thoughts, become neutral and even passive, and wait for a response. Isn't that what we do when we are there for a friend? We need to do the same thing with the same courtesy with our spirit guides. That instant popping of thought will signal to you that you are receiving a response. You gave yourself time to receive and time to listen in a different way. Most of the time, listening is really a telepathic pop of information.

### Symbols

Symbols are images that represent focused information. Symbols are everywhere in our culture. They are in business logos and on business cards. They are in everything from board games to billboards along a highway. Symbols also appear in the language of Spirit. Spirit can give the receiver a volume of knowledge in one image. For instance, I often see eyes during a reading. Eyes are said to be the windows of the soul, and I glean a great deal of information from the eyes that I see, where they appear, how they appear, and what action or non-action they are taking.

Spirit will tend to offer symbols because they give you such a volume of information in an instant. For example, if the image of a hammer were to appear during a medical intuition scan, I would notice the location and what it's doing. Does it appear around or within the person's body or their energy field? Is it lying on the floor, or is it being used to pound something or as a weapon? Is it being used to pry open something or to remove a nail from wood?

Symbols can be images of objects, scenes as if in a movie, or patterns. A symbol could appear in your mind's eye as a mandala, an animal, a house, a mountain, or a knight's armor. There is absolutely no end to the symbols that may come to you and no end to the meaning they represent. Simply tell the person of the symbol, where it is located, and the action or lack of action it has. Inquire what meaning it has for the person that you are scanning. Allow them to offer the deeper meaning first before you offer its potential meaning. You do not need to figure it out for them.

### Pictures

There is an old saying that one picture says a thousand words, and that is the truth. As you delve into the human body, you might see, in your mind's eye, an entire scene stretching out before you. It might appear as a painting or a photo or even an event unfolding before your eyes. Take note of all the elements and all the components within that picture. For instance, if the picture in your mind is a group of people, notice everything about the people. What are the expressions on their faces? What emotions are you picking up? How are they standing and what proximity are they to the client? Are the people in the image standing shoulder to shoulder? Are they standing separate or are some standing together while one stands to the side?

Let's say a picture popped into your mind as you scan a person's lungs. If the picture in your mind is a landscape, what components stand out to you? What might a landscape of an early spring, full of bright, new green color, tell you about their lungs? How would you get a different impression if the landscape was of deep winter and everything was frozen over?

Can you sense the importance in noticing the details in the image? Can you sense that the details are giving you immediate, significant information about the functioning of the lungs? Of course, each of these examples has a completely different feel. Now adjust your initial impressions of each image and what they tell you about a person's lungs. It could possibly be a springtime of new healing in the lungs or difficulty in breathing and feeling as if the lungs are frozen and struggling to expand. Simply describe to your client what you see in the picture. Your client will know what it means.

### Body Sensations within the Practitioner
Sometimes you will physically sense the struggles of your clients within your own body. It is imperative that you understand you are not picking up the illness and making it your own. Be aware that as your sensitivity heightens, you will sense the energy signatures of another person's illness within your own body. For instance, I felt great one day as I began a phone reading. The moment I touched in with this person's energy field, I noticed that my own throat felt swollen on the right side and seemed sore. I was not getting their illness. I was picking up energetic signals from the energy of another. The signals in your own body are simply waves of information about the client. Again, you are not getting their illness. You are receiving information.

I often give mini readings at psychic expos because I find that it hones my skills and it often helps people who would not ordinarily sit for a lengthy assessment. A delightful woman with a huge smile on her face sat down in front of me. As we greeted each other, my heart instantly began beating way too fast and felt as if was going to jump out of my chest. I said, "You are having a lot of strong heart palpitations, are you not?" The shocked look on her face told me I was correct.

She responded, "I have been feeling them for months now. No one knows! I have not told anyone about it!" I explained what the palpitations might be about and told her that she must go to a physician for a medical evaluation as soon as possible.

I have also felt the pressure of a potential heart attack in my own chest during a medical intuitive scan for a client. I knew my body was not feeling that pressure just prior to the reading, which told me it was a signal from my client. Your psychic sensors are picking up the energetic signals but not the illness. An intuitive signal is not the same as receiving the illness.

The best way to know what is happening is to know your own

body, especially just prior to a medical intuitive session. You will be able to tell the difference and your clients will confirm those particular symptoms. In a commanding way within your mind, say to Spirit, "I thank you for the signal and information. It is not mine; out of me now." Feel that you are pushing the signal right out of your body.

### Sounds

You might think you are imagining sounds around the person you are scanning. You know that the sounds are not in the room you are physically sitting in and they are not coming from the building or from outside of the building. You will realize that the sounds are coming from the energy field of the person sitting before you. For example, as you connect with a client you might get vague or even loud impressions of people yelling and arguing. Notice the location of the sounds. In other words, in what proximity are the sounds to the client? During one episode, I heard yelling coming from behind my client, so I described that impression and told her that the fighting was all around her and quite loud. She agreed that her entire family was constantly fighting, and she felt she was at the center of the fighting but did not know how to change what was happening.

In another example, you might hear a gentle, sweet sound throughout a client's entire body except for his or her heart. The heart might seem out of sync or out of tune from the rest of the body. What might that mean to you and your client? In this case it might signify that this person is not living their heart's desire or the heart is physically stressed and overworked.

Some areas on your client's body may sound very quiet while other areas may sound quite active. What if you begin to hear the vague sound of a fire alarm? Do not discount it as too weird. Inform your client. The person might tell you that they live near a fire station and the alarm is causing them a great deal of stress. Take note of your client's body to discern where that particular stress is centering and let them know about it.

Sounds and vibrational tones seem to be the most ignored sensory pathway of information for the medical intuitive. Begin to notice if you are a sound-sensitive intuitive. Utilize that sense when it happens and use it to assist others. Do not push it aside thinking it is not important or a coincidence.

### Smells and Tastes
You might be able to pick up smells, fragrances, and odors of certain conditions within the person you are assisting. Do not underestimate smells and think it is just your imagination. Smells, while usually physical in nature, can also be a form of energetic information about another person. One example might be a sudden awareness of cigarette or cigar smoke when you scan someone's lungs. The person I am thinking of declared that they had not smoked for five years, yet the energetic vibration of cigarettes remained within her body.

I have picked up the bitter smell of chemicals in a farmer who handled herbicides and fertilizers all of his life. There is a certain bitter, metallic, chemical odor and taste with people who have received or are receiving chemotherapy. One man who had this energetic signal told me that his chemotherapy happened six years prior to our reading. I have been aware of a thickness in my mouth and a taste that is slightly sweet for people who are diabetic. The stronger the thickness in my mouth and the stronger the taste of sugar, the more severe the diabetes is.

Allow your body to give you these subtle energetic indicators. Like the intuitive information in the form of sounds, smells and taste also carry energetic signals that often give you vital evidence for the person who has come to you for help. Remember that you are picking up indicators and not contracting someone's illness.

### Focused Attention
As I began a medical intuition scan one day, I began, as usual, to look at the energy field in general and then focus on this person's head in my usual process of going from head to toe. In spite of my

determination to follow a logical path through the human body, I kept skipping entire sections of the body and was powerfully drawn to this person's hands and primarily his right hand. I kept bringing myself back in an attempt to follow my usual pattern of scanning, only to be brought back to his hands. It was as if I was forcefully pushed to the hands.

Finally, a light bulb went off in my head, and I realized that this man's hands were the priority for this reading. When I stopped fighting the guidance my medical intuitive guides were giving me, I told him what I was getting about his hands. He exclaimed, "Yes, that is why I came to you!" The entire reading was about his hands.

When your attention is being pulled to a certain area of your client's body, go with the pull. There is a powerful reason for why we are pulled to a specific portion of the body. Please do not try to follow a certain pattern for the medical intuitive session. You are the only one who thinks there needs to be a pattern. Your guides and your clients may have other ideas. Your clients and your guidance is the priority.

The more you turn it over to Spirit, the more direction you will receive. We need to be aware of divine direction and follow its guidance. When Spirit wants you to pay attention to certain aspects during a medical intuition session, you need to pay attention and go with their guidance. Sometimes they will become more forceful if you ignore it. Spirit guiding your work and your focus will always be clearer than we can ever be alone.

Throughout the remainder of this book, I ask that you become more and more aware of the pathways that intuitive information comes to you. I also ask that you look for new pathways that you have not noticed in the past.

Document this awareness about yourself now.

**Your Client's Guides**

The medical intuitive practitioner is not the only one with spirit guidance. When your client walks into a session with you, an average of two to five deceased loved ones might come in with them. This person will have a spirit guide or two or even a group of guides with them. While these guides may not be specialists in the way we have been discussing, they are clients' personal specialists in their life, their death, and beyond. Every person has guides that remain with him or her forever and guides who come during particular times in a person's life.

Spiritualists teach that we have five primary guides focused on different areas of life. For example, there is a joy guide to help bring happiness into our life. We have other guides who are teachers, healers, and spiritual development guides who assist us with different aspects of life. Some people also feel powerfully drawn to angels and have sensitive experiences with the angelic realm.

Elizabeth was eager to participate in my assessment. She was very open, and it was easy to perceive her energy. I was receiving some general information that was informative for her but not really remarkable until I entered her chest and her heart. Layers and layers of protection greeted me like the thin dough of a pie crust. As I described this to her, I told her that they seemed to be placed there little by little over time. A little protection developed during one painful situation, and then later a little more protection developed on top of it. Over time, those thin layers became a thick barrier that prevented energy from coming in or leaving. As I described the protective layers around her, she relaxed a little. When she relaxed the protection around her, thousands of tiny, hot, sharp, needle-like bolts of energy shot out of her. A huge release of old anger and hurt began to happen.

I then moved on to Elizabeth's abdomen and found a huge, gaping hole from the edge of her diaphragm all the way to her second chakra. Suddenly a Native American male stood at my side. I watched him place his hands into the darkness of her body's hole. He began to literally scoop out a substance that appeared like dull cottage cheese. He scooped the congealed, blackened energy out and placed it beyond my visual field. I remained quiet, respectful, and observant as I waited. As he dug into her belly, a clear purple beam of light shot into the gaping hole. Elizabeth's spirit guide then firmly voiced, "No one has your power but you. I am scooping out your denial. Now you have to do this yourself." I memorized these words so I could relay them to her. He went on, "We are this far away (sweeping his arms far apart) because you are not attending to Spirit."

As he faded away, I immediately noticed an older couple in spirit. I described them to Elizabeth, and she confirmed that they were her grandparents on her mother's side. They did not seem to have anything to add to her Native American guide's wisdom, but they wanted her to know they supported her. Elizabeth's spirit guide performed this dramatic healing as two of her deceased loved ones supported her. I was only a witness so she could receive the information as accurately as possible. I had very little to do with this intimate restorative development, yet she remembered and described it to me twelve years later.

### Essential Point:
*You are the communication link between the physical and the non-physical.*

June's medical intuitive assessment came in many visually clear images. Immediately, the glowing presence of an angel with broad outstretched wings appeared, as if it might take off at any second even though it just arrived. It seemed to hover around the top of June's head, rising up from her crown and third eye. The high energy seemed to release excess heat and prickles from her brain. A Native American female then stood on June's right side. She bowed to June in a respectful gesture. I instantly began to see forests, animals, and birds. One tree had large, beautiful eyes smiling out. The spirit asked me to tell June, "Your wisdom is as old as the trees. Use it and do not doubt." I told June these words and informed her that this spirit guide emphasized the words "use it." June said she knew exactly what that statement was about.

You will naturally see spirit guides during your sessions. Medical intuitive practitioners are able to witness these guides performing healings and giving profound messages during readings. It is vital that we as practitioners express every detail to the person we are working with. While we are not interpreting the content of what we pick up intuitively, we are communicating for Spirit.

It is essential that you memorize the experience as it unfolds and commit to accurately quoting the guide's message. Quoting for Spirit is different than offering an interpretation. You are a vital link for all who participate in a medical intuitive process. We are working for Spirit as much as we are working for our loved ones and our clients. Remember that these experiences will constantly seems as if you are making it all up, but it is totally real. Allow yourself to access this valuable information and proudly be the communication link between the physical and the non-physical.

# Chapter Seven

## Prepare for Auras and Chakras

### Failing to Perceive Auras

If you think you cannot see auras, then you definitely will not perceive them. First you must acknowledge that sensing energy is a fundamental sensual ability of humans. We are wired to perceive from the physical world, and we are wired to perceive the non-physical world too. Our intuitive instincts often kept us alive in the caves of ancient times and throughout our personal history. You must now accept that you are simply going to perceive energy fields. Immediately accept it and understand this is an innate ability you can practice everywhere and with everyone.

You will find it is easier to practice sensing the aura when people are pumped up or excited. Practice with people who are presenting a speech or performing before others. Look above a group of people who are singing together, such as a choir, and look for the energy that is building as they sing. Watch a teacher present a lecture. People who are performing before others tend to emit a higher level of energy at those times and as a result, it is easier to sense the energy field around them.

As you begin to practice perceiving auras, do not try hard to look for color! Look only for a thickness in the air around the head and shoulders of people. The air will appear slightly denser an inch or so from the body. You might detect a faint line where the air seems to go from thicker to thinner a couple of inches from the head.

Remember, the aura is extremely subtle because it is non-physical. It is not solid in any way, shape, or form, and it will not sit there waiting for you. It is wispy, flowing, shooting outward and shrinking back. It is completely transparent. It is alive and lively. Do not expect it to look physical or thick or stable or solid. Every thought changes this energy field. Every emotion changes it instantly as well.

As you begin to practice sensing auras using the steps outlined below, do not focus on seeing colors. Focus only on seeing wispy, changing fleeting movement. One second you think you see it and the next minute it is gone.

**Essential Point:**
*The aura is alive, moving, and transparent.*
*It does not hold still.*

**Basic Steps to Perceive Auras**

1. Practice with a person who is energetic and feeling well because their aura will be larger and more vibrant. Have that person stand near a smooth wall of a neutral color. Change the lighting so there are no shadows around the person.

2. Remember to let the imagination wave flow through your mind and allow the spirit mind to feel daydreamlike. Do not try hard to do this. Do not use any effort.

3. Allow your eyes to un-focus. Let them feel lazy or heavy. If you wear glasses, take them off while you practice. The un-focusing will be helpful.

4. Do not actively look, but instead allow your eyes to passively sense the transparent thickness in the air about one to three inches beyond the edge of the person's skin or clothing. Look only for the thickness of the aura around the shoulders and head. Remember: lazy eyes, unfocused eyes, no effort.

5. Again, do not try to see the color but instead imagine a

color as you look toward that person. Simply make it up for now. "If I was seeing a color around you now it would be _____."

6. Focus on the feel of that color. What would it feel like if you put your fingers into it? What emotions come about as you sense that particular color?

7. Ask your practice person to focus on a certain color by thinking and feeling that color. Ask the person to not tell you what color they are thinking. Ask that person to feel as if they are pushing that same color out past their skin. With lazy eyes, simply notice the air around this person.

8. With lazy eyes, playfully experience the aura.

9. Repeat this process with as many people as you can. Practice on your pets as well.

Describe your awareness with each person in your journal.

## The Aura Surges with Information

Each section of this book builds on the last section and prepares the reader for the next. An examination of the aura is our next step. A medical intuitive scan is like reading an intimate biography. The outer auric field is similar to opening the book's cover and reading the introduction. Moving into the physical body is the same as reading each chapter in one's life story. Most medical intuitives assess another human in a similar order. They might immediately notice the general auric field, then the chakras, and then past the skin into the physical body.

The aura is the visible portion of the human soul. The energy and form of the individual soul is much larger than the human body can contain beneath the boundaries of the skin. The soul is a force of electromagnetic frequencies, and those frequencies flow and surge in constant undulating waves of aliveness. Your soul energy ripples in rising and falling swells throughout the body and it also ripples in waves throughout one's life. The skin is not like rubber insulation that confines the electricity going to a table lamp or the TV. The soul extends outward across the earth plane and upward into the heavens of the cosmos.

### Essential Point:
*A medical intuitive scan is like reading
an intimate biography.*

Michael Newton explains in his book *Journey of Souls* that people tend to bring only a portion of their soul energy with them into their physical incarnations. When I was using hypnosis for regressions and for life between lives regressions, I frequently heard the same information from my clients as well. They often describe that a portion of their individuality always remains in the spirit realm while the remainder of their soul energy dwells within a human body.

### Essential Point:
*When you see an aura, you are witnessing a soul.*

Recurring thoughts and emotions either build or distress the energy field. The aura becomes and holds the most prominent positive or the most prominent negative vibrations. These vibrations emanate from our past lives and from our current lives, creating our most prominent possibilities for the future.

I know of a family of three sisters who are in their seventies and eighties. I personally know one of the sisters; she is bright, positive, and full of life. Her two sisters have lived their lives in a different way, hating each other since they were teens. The fighting has been constant throughout the years. My friend is saddened for them because they have refused to have any contact with each other. Their lives have been filled with hate while my friend's life has been full of love. My friend is a physically healthy woman and both of her sisters have been placed in different nursing homes for dementia.

Another dear friend offers an example of the effects of hate on the physical body. This woman is openly full of rage and hate, blaming everyone in her path for all of her miseries. This woman is also in a nursing home. And guess what? She is also in a secured dementia unit! The energy of relentless hate affected these women's bodies, their minds, and their lives.

As you enter into a human's energy field, you are entering into their entire story. You will experience the good, the bad, and the ugly. You will perceive their blissful moments and their agony. You are experiencing the electrical nature of the eternal soul incorporated within the human body, flooded with thoughts, emotions, and powerful beliefs.

The aura also is a pattern. This pattern encompasses the entire scope of each human, from the subatomic particles that make up the physical human body to the expanse of the heavens. While physical and mental health is reflected in each moment of the human aura, it also holds the unceasing story that is created, generated, and influenced by many other factors. The following factors also influence the body and aura and will certainly come up during a session:

- Choices and decisions
- Genetic heritage
- Energy patterns of our ancestors
- Upbringing
- Parent's lifestyle
- Food and nutrition
- Relationships
- Earth's electromagnetic field
- Current life experiences
- Current life history
- Past lives
- The intergalactic realm

You are not in control. Do not attempt to control the reading by focusing on each influence. The more prominent information will naturally flow into your awareness. Let the information guide you. During a medical intuitive session, you will not receive information from every single item listed above. All intuitives tend to access the most prominent components that are affecting that person, positively and negatively, in the moment. Sometimes a past life will rush into the forefront of your awareness. Sometimes a genetic factor of the person's ancestors will draw your attention. With another person, you might pick up that the earth's energy is placing stress on the individual.

There are certainly no limits in what might explode into your intuitive awareness during a session. Hopefully, this list of influences will help you understand you are not crazy when something strange jumps into your awareness during an assessment. If you suddenly think about the sun's solar flares negatively affecting someone, do not discount it. If you begin to see a model of DNA as you give a medical intuitive assessment, take it into account and share the information you get. If you find yourself on another planet during an intuitive reading, discuss it with your client. Go with anything that comes into your awareness.

**Essential Point:**
*You are not in control.*
***Do not attempt to control the reading.***

The following is a description of the aura of a woman that I met in 2003. Her aura blushed in pinkish purple all around the top of her head, including both right and left side of her brain and her third eye. The lower portion of her face appeared as a faint rainbow. Everything looked quite positive. I scanned down to her shoulders where I found the right shoulder tight and tense while the left shoulder emerged with hot balls of prickly, dark red anger. Some of the red hung deep into the muscle and some floated a few inches about the shoulder in the outer auric field.

This woman's heart was bright yellow and seemed to be the shape of an open flower with large petals. Her abdomen had tiny little holes in it, but yellow light twinkled outward through the small openings. Her lower abdomen had threads of dark, ruddy-looking orange. Her legs appeared equally balanced in brighter orange flowing upward. All this information came from the aura's vibrations in the first few minutes of the reading.

In as little as three minutes, a medical intuitive can sense a wealth of information from an individual's auric field. Its features are determined by the level of the person's vitality in that moment as well as one's immediate thoughts, emotions, life themes, and patterns in one's current life. Each person is a multifaceted, complicated, unique being. The assessment I made in three minutes is only a general outline in an eternal story.

I have compiled the aura table following this section describing each color's associated emotional and thought qualities. The descriptive words include both positive and negative characteristics for that color's vibration. Our emotions as well as our thoughts emanate energetic vibrations and those vibrations can be visualized by humans within the light spectrum that our eyes are able to discern.

You might already be asking, "How do I know if I am seeing a positive trait or its negative element?" I determine positive and negative traits by noticing the characteristics of each color. Negative thoughts and emotions actually radiate in short, slow, choppy waves of energy. The happier, more pleasant thoughts and emotions appear in fine, smooth, and fast wave frequencies. The more negative the emotion, the thicker, darker or muddier the color will be. The more positive the emotion, the lighter and more glowing the color will be.

## Color Interpretation of the Aura

There is a distinctive intelligence within all energy and a great amount of information is within the finer details. When we truly notice the subtle details of anything, we allow more information in. Look for these finer details in the visible aura and the vibratory levels of color because a great deal of information is there for the medical intuitive.

**Essential Point:**
*Subtle details of your perceptions hold the information.*

On the next page is a quick color table for you to utilize during your practice sessions. Remember, this is only a guideline. Always make sure you adjust your awareness to the person you are working with. In other words, always acknowledge the individual and how the color vibrations reflect individuality in that moment. The color interpretations are not set in stone. It provides only a guideline for you to begin your medical intuition journey perceiving energetic information from colors in the energy field. Each person is unique and you are unique also. Perceive each aura based on the individual that you are working with.

Notice that the descriptive words following each color include positive and negative qualities.

Your accuracy as a medical intuitive will escalate by examining all the subtle, priceless details along with the general intuitive information that comes to you.

| Color Interpretation Table | |
|---|---|
| Red | cellular health, energy, high temper, movement, extroversion |
| Light Red | nervous, impulsive, passion, eroticism, sexuality, love |
| Dark Red | willpower, masculinity, rage, courage, suffering, leadership |
| Pink | femininity, longings, sensitivity, emotional, softness |
| Orange | active intelligence, confident, expressive, warmth, joy of life, sex |
| Orange-Red | taking action, pride, vanity, idealism, desire |
| Yellow | sharp intellect, quick wit, industrious |
| Dark Yellow | timid, thrift, restrictions, control needs |
| Gold | devotion, higher inspiration, meditative state, authority, creative |
| Forest Green | abundance, harvest, rich growth |
| Green | growth, change, nature, devotion, neutral state, healing, harmony |
| Light Green | sympathy, direct, possible deceit or lying |
| Blue | introversion, solitude, truth, devotion to spirit, wisdom, prayer, writing |
| Light Blue | softness, religious, reserved, struggle to mature |
| Indigo | healing ability, morality, immersed in work, spiritual, mediumship |
| Turquoise | giving love to others in a healing capacity, expansion |
| Lavender | mysticism, magic, overbearing, obsessions |
| Violet | intuition, art, creativity, supernatural, imagination |
| Clear White | eternal, forever, god-like |
| Milky White | spirituality, higher consciousness, physical pain |
| Silver | mother love without conditions |
| Black | protection, shielding, detached from senses, meditative |
| Gray | duty, karma, not taking action, depressed |
| Brown | egotism, addiction, dis-ease, earthiness, unloving |

### Location of Auric Colors

Notice the location that each color vibration appears. This awareness will give you more detailed information about the individual you are assisting. Understanding the common meaning of each color and associating it with a certain area of the body is a key factor in your assessment. For example, a certain color appearing in the muscles of the upper back will provide a great deal of information. But if that same color appears in the client's liver it will probably have a different meaning. A grayish yellow in the left side of the upper back will have a completely different meaning than that same grayish yellow hovering within the gall-bladder.

Making a connection with the meaning of each color and where it appears in and around the client's body brings a more precise understanding of what is going on. (We will identify the significance of the various parts of the human anatomy in Chapter Eight.)

### Shape

The general shape of the auric colors around the body will immediately inform you about the vitality of the person you are working with. It will also tell you about the vitality of different areas and organs of the body. You will immediately know what areas of the body are low or high in energy. In some areas, the aura may stretch into the room, while in a different area, the aura may extend only an inch from the body. While one area may appear low, another area of the body might appear highly energized.

Some areas may jut out in spikes, while others might appear smooth. Spikes signify sharp, critical thoughts while a softer edge denotes a softer attitude. Look at the overall aura for dips, concaved areas, spikes or soft, round areas, or even holes. Remember that the aura constantly fluctuates, clearly apparent in one area for a moment then gone the next. In general, a healthy aura will tend to be uniform.

## Size

While the general shape of the aura and the colors will give you immediate impressions, the size of the energetic field will disclose the extent of health or disease in that area. The size will often tell you about the severity of the situation or the extent of an emotional response. It will distinguish the volume or expanse of the situation, positive or negative. For example, recognizing a color radiating in a huge twelve-inch column from someone's chest will give you different information than if that same color is witnessed as a pinpoint of light.

Size will often inform you about the intensity of illness or emotion. If you perceive a certain section of the aura hovering close to the skin, the situation is either new or the person is trying to hide the emotion. If it seems to extend out beyond your own intuitive vision it has probably been there quite some time or the person is making sure that everyone knows about their thoughts and emotions.

## Transparency, Sparkle

A general guideline that I use is this: If it isn't transparent and shimmery, it is not healthy or positive. Healthy auric colors exuding outward, past the skin, are generally transparent and film-like, allowing the intuitive to visualize the wall or the lamp behind the client. In other words, you should be able to see the aura and beyond that the wall and the lamp. If the aura is thick or darkened, this signifies something has been there for a long time or unhealthiness. The transparency or the lack of transparency is very informative if you notice this detail.

## Density

If the energy field is not transparent, what is it? The energy will naturally appear denser as you perceive the aura closer to the body because it is emanating from the body in a slower vibration. The aura will naturally appear thinner as it extends farther from the body because it is less physical and vibrates faster and finer.

Because the aura is the soul and living energy, it also emanates inside the physical body as well. A healthy energy field, deep within the human body, will appear translucent and shimmery, but the colors might seem denser and less transparent because you are witnessing it on a more physical level. Organs, muscle, tissue, and bones are dense, and the energy can appear denser but still be healthy.

As a medical intuitive, you will notice this natural variation of a person's aura from dense to fine. You will also be assessing internal organs and areas that are not light and bright. When the aura in a certain area is thicker and less bright than the other portions of the human body, it will tell you that the energy is not flowing there. That lack of brightness will signify a potential illness or an illness that has already manifested.

You can assess those areas and organs by projecting your laser beam deeper into the person's body. There are thousands of ways the human body and the energy field may appear to you. For example, it might seem as if you are looking through plastic food wrap, a thin piece of cloth, or even a thick blanket. The thicker the color, the longer the situation has been developing. Thick and dull or dark will signify a struggle, a potential illness or an existing illness.

Scan the air around the individual looking for areas that seem thicker or thinner. For instance, as John sat in my chair telling me about the enduring conflict with his three siblings, the aura around his head looked gelatinous—in other words, thicker. It was also not as transparent as it could be. The thickness and decreased transparency denoted the heaviness he felt about the ongoing struggle to understand his siblings.

With some people, it may feel as if you are pushing through glue or even wet cement. Notice if the density is in one area or if it is over the entire body. A thick aura may consist of one layer or many layers. It might confirm the person has built up a protection around them, but it can also signify a long-term problem. Generally, the thicker it feels or appears, the longer it has been there.

Thickness, however, does not always signify illness. For example, a thick but bright yellow all on the left side of someone's head may mean that the person tends to live more in their logical mind and they do not recognize the creative aspect of life. In my experience, a combination of thick and less bright denotes struggles in that area of the body.

## Cloudiness/Muddiness

The specific shade of color will give you even more information about which emotion is prevalent. The color might appear more opaque, dull, or gloomy, as if some degree of gray has been added to the color. Gray shades often signify a level of depression. A heavy cloudiness will denote a heaviness of emotions. The area of the body it appears in will ultimately give you even more information. For example, a grayish orange throughout the solar plexus might tell you that the person struggles with confidence while that same strange color throughout the first chakra might tell you that this person struggles with sexual expression or has been abused.

Muddy shades of color seem to offer different information than cloudiness. If a color is muddy it implies there are tints of murky darkness, as if brown has been added to the primary color. The muddier a color is, the longer a situation has gone on. An example here would be my perception of anger. I see anger as a muddy, maroon red. The darker the muddy red, the older or more stagnant the anger is for that person. The longer that person has been holding onto a heavy emotion, the muddier it is.

## Color Combinations

You may be perceiving colors such as turquoise or pinks. Turquoise is actually the combination of green and blue, and pink is red infused with white. When you see colors mixing, you are literally witnessing a combination of qualities of the individual colors (see the color table). When turquoise appears to be more blue, it might inform you that this person spends a great deal of time in prayer (blue), especially regarding healing (green) for self or others. Blue equates communication with spirit while greens denote healing.

Another example is bright, candy apple red. That color vibration will inform you that the person has a great deal of cellular health while at the same time feels a feminine sensitivity about an issue. Pink combines physical vitality of red with white of sensitivity to create a vibration of unconditional love.

### Movement/No Movement

Energetic movement gives the medical intuitive a great deal of information. One can learn about a medical situation by feeling or visualizing the strength and vigor of the movement within specific areas of the body. The key is in the energetic force or lack of force in·and around the body.

Movement will vary from sluggish to zooming or somewhere in between. The movement, or lack of it, is very telling and will give you even more information. If muddy red is flashing outward from a person's throat or mouth, you will know they are currently expressing or recently expressed anger. If that same muddy red is sitting still in the throat, you will understand this person is holding it in, pushing it down, or may not even be aware of anger at all.

The medical intuitive may also pick up a tremulous, wave-like energy. Over the years I have come to associate this waviness, especially over the head or the abdomen, as anxiety. It seems that we humans either hold anxiety in our heads or we take it in the gut. I have also found that a great deal of anxiety tends to sit in the upper chest just below the base of the throat.

When you describe tremors to clients, they will agree with you that they do indeed feel anxiety in that particular area of their body. They will have a lump in their throat and can hardly swallow or their stomach tightens and they cannot eat. The human body really takes a hit when anxiety focuses in certain areas. The tremulous area, however, will give you very important information to discuss with your client during your session.

The aura is not just the energy that extends beyond the skin of humans. The aura is the energetic, eternal essence and life form of one's being. You can follow the aura from its finer outer levels down past the skin and into the muscle and fiber of each person. The aura permeates each organ, gland, tissue, and bone, all the way to the spinal column.

**Essential Point:**
*The aura is the energetic, eternal essence
and life form of one's being.*

### Direction of Movement

If a color is floating outward, the person is likely emitting their energy in a normal, everyday manner. However, if the color is jetting outward like a rocket, the person is actively feeling or actively interrelating in the situation at hand. Energy rushing outward like a fire hose might signify that the person is losing too much energy and may not be able to receive enough energy to replenish their vitality.

Stay alert regarding the direction of energetic movement. If the energy seems to be entering the individual from the outside inward, you may conclude they are receiving something in life. If the movement inward feels chaotic and rough, it could signify that someone is fighting with your client.

A thick dense energy sitting on your client's shoulder may tell you that the client is taking on too much responsibility or other people's baggage. In other words, when we try to assume the responsibilities of other people's lives we are also altering our own energy field. When we try to fix everything for our loved ones we actually carry the burden around for them.

The volume of the color, as it enters or as it leaves the body, will determine the positive or negative strength of the situation as it occurs. If it appears thin as a pencil, then the situation is either new or does not affect the client too terribly. If the movement feels or appears like a fire hose, you will know that the effect is more dramatic for the client. The color and the shade of the color then adds information to your assessment.

## Sound

The visual experience of each color is caused by a vibration of energy that touches the retina of the eye. While we see energy in colors, the energy of each color also creates a very subtle sound. A hummingbird's wings create one sound as it hovers over the feeder and another sound when it fights off another hummingbird trying to approach the same feeder. One rate of wing movement generates one particular sound and another rate of movement creates a slightly different sound.

Some medical intuitives have a finely tuned sense of sound. Each color will have a distinctive tone. The sounds may be musical, but more commonly each color has a certain tone. It is important to distinguish the quality of the tones. It may sound out of tune, flat, tinny, dull, or the tone may be pleasing like a hum of a hummingbird's wings. Stretch your mind and play around with the sounds of color.

## Leaks

Look for leaks in the energy field. Leaks are created from a physical or an emotional trauma. The trauma can be caused by something as simple as a tooth being worked on to being struck by an abuser. Someone may have a leak in their aura from a family member or a friend saying something deeply painful. Leaks will feel or look like a string of tiny to large-sized bubbles floating up and out of the body. Imagine looking into a pan of water just before it begins to boil and you will see little strings of bubbles rising upward. That is the look and also the physical sensation of leaks. The size of the leak depends on how severe the person perceives the trauma to be emotionally or how severe the trauma was physically.

## Pain

As you enter into the aura of another person, a sense of physical pain may be evident. You may become aware of pain because the thought of it jumped into your thoughts or you might see the word "pain" in your mind. You might momentarily receive the information as a signal in your own body. When I sense someone's physical pain in my own body, I say a word of thanks for receiving the message but I also say, "It is not mine. Out of me now." Notice if the pain seems to sit there or if there is movement to the pain. If the pain seems to shoot outward, it often signifies the person is releasing it. If it sits there in one place, the body may be holding onto it.

Notice the quality of the pain. Tiny, hot needles may be a symptom of being "needled" by someone in life. It may also mean physical inflammation in the area it appears. Long, stabbing pain often comes out of people's heads or their hearts. They might feel as if they have been stabbed by someone important in life. Achiness or even waves of ache often comes from the organ of the heart or the heart chakra, which literally denotes heartache. Physical achiness often comes from joints or muscles.

Again, if you are not clear on the origin of pain, ask for guidance. Take note of the area of the body the pain is coming from and the deeper meanings of the chakra that is nearby. Be aware of your thoughts, your "knowing," and physical sensations that you feel. As you learn and perfect your medical assessments, you will know if the pain is emotionally or physically based. You can also ask your spirit guide for clarification.

### Cool/Hot Areas

Look for and sense the general temperature of your client's energy field. After noticing the general temperature of the person, search for areas that seem hotter or cooler than the general temperature of the rest of the body. Excess heat in an area may signify inflammation, physical illness, emotional turmoil, or an over-worked internal organ. A very cool area might imply extremely low energy, a thick energetic shield covering the area, scar tissue, or constricted energy flow. Notice what chakra is near the area where the temperature seems different. Each chakra also represents certain energy signatures that correspond with certain energetic meanings. Ask your spirit guide to clearly tell you if this issue is physically, mentally, or spiritually created.

### Thin/Bulging

Sometimes the size of the aura appears to be consistent around the body but in one or more places it has an indentation, as if it has been scooped out. That dip or thinness in the field signifies a loss of energy or a constricted flow of energy in that area. It represents a struggle of some type that has affected the body's performance. For example, the person may have lost some of their essence by giving it away, or it was taken by an abuser

Take note of that area, and what organ and which chakra is nearby. A thin aura may tell you that the person is exhausted and depleted. A thin aura will feel like you are struggling to get through film or plastic food wrap. Ask your spirit guide to clearly tell you if this issue is physically, mentally, or spiritually created.

You may notice that the aura feels as if it has an outward bulge that far exceeds the other portions of the person's aura. I listened to a man describe to a small group of his friends that he was madly in love with a woman. As he talked, the energy bulged outward from his chest in a rosy-pink color. If he had been describing anger about this woman, a rush of dark muddy red would have flowed outward. Any deeply felt emotion, positive or negative, will quickly spill or bulge outward. On a positive note, a bulging energy around the heart, for example, might also show that the person's heart chakra is wide open and they give a great deal to life or to other people. This type of bulge will feel positive and light, not heavy or dense.

There is a distinction between a rush of energy and a quiet, sluggish bulge of energy that just sits there in the auric field. While this rush of energy signifies immediate emotions, a bulge signifies other possibilities. A bulge may signal an older, long-lasting emotion or unresolved issue that has been building up over the years. It may denote some type of physical trauma. It may also show you that the area, organ, or chakra is overworked.

For example, the aura of a diabetic's pancreas may bulge due to the illness overtaxing it.

## Examples of Auric Colors

One auric color example that I love to discuss is the vibratory color of telling lies. Lying appears as the color of baby crap. If you are a parent, you will know what I mean. The bowel movement of young babies is a combination of brown, olive green, and murky yellow. One day a woman was talking to me about renting a property that I owned. "Baby crap" shot out the sides of her neck in pencil-thick rays of energy about eight inches in length. Based on the discussion above, what do you make of this description? Think about it before you move on for my explanation.

Mud brown, the base color, is thick and dense, so it depicts disease or heaviness and a strong ego justifying the lies within their mind. The yellow is not bright like the sun but murky. Yellow is the vibration of the intellect and active thinking, which might tell you the person is calculating and aware that they are purposely lying. The green is a light lime shade but also overcast and shadowy. A muddy lime green denotes deceit. Put this all together for the vibrational signature of consciously lying and feeling justified in doing so. Needless to say that woman did not become my tenant!

Let's talk about the color vibration of cancer. Every single time I have come across cancer it looks exactly the same. It appears as shiny, black, liquid tar that looks like hot asphalt being poured on a road. I have also perceived it as a sparkler spurting in all directions. I see this tar-like substance with people who are already diagnosed with cancer or people who are soon diagnosed with cancer. You must look at all the factors or size, shape, thickness, and location of the black tar. When it shows itself as sparks shooting out in all directions, it is a fast-growing cancer.

I have never witnessed cancer energy in the outer aura. I have only witnessed it inside of the person's physical body. If the person already knows they have cancer, I verbally describe its location and if it seems to have spread. I describe the size and thickness of the darkness. I offer some insights about the emotions and old, old thoughts that possibly fed into this disease.

A strong reminder: If the person is unaware that they have cancer, you cannot diagnose unless you are a licensed physician. I *never* say the word cancer, but I do describe, describe, and describe some more. I give precise details of how it looks and feels, and its location. I calmly mention that this particular area of the body seems stressed and needs medical attention. I sometimes ask the client to call his or her doctor that day.

So far, each of my clients have followed through with medical attention and each one of them was diagnosed with some form of cancer in the location that I perceived it in. I, however, did not diagnose the problem. I described in specific detail how it appeared or felt or the knowing that came into my awareness. Do not terrify the person with your own fear. Be professional, matter-of-fact, and firm about what you perceive. Be the professional in all situations, even the situation of cancer.

No clear color is bad, not even black. There is a positive side of the black spectrum because it also appears in various degrees of density, transparency, shade, etc. In the example of cancer, a heavy, asphalt-like depth of black signifies dramatic illness. Black, on the other end of this spectrum, denotes protection. Black is often a covering or a shield protecting something vulnerable. I see many, many black shields over people's hearts for example. It does not mean they have cancer of the heart, nor does it mean they have black-hearted intent. It means they have suffered from emotional experiences and have decided to put up a barrier between their emotional center and the rest of the world.

**Essential Point:**
*No clear color is bad, not even black.*

Each time you pick up color within the aura, carefully take note of all the aspects that define its character. Notice the location of the color around the body. Notice if the color is moving or stagnant. Be aware of its sheen or its lackluster, its clarity or murkiness, thickness or density, the movement and volume of movement and the direction it takes. Also be aware of its size and shape.

All of these details provide you with detailed information. These distinctive traits are specific energy signatures, and each signature defines the emotional makeup that is currently present. Your ability to perceive the auric field in detail will greatly amplify your ability as an accurate medical intuitive.

Now that we have discussed visualizing color, let's look at other significant factors regarding the more physical impressions that you might feel in someone's aura.

## A Medical Intuitive's Chakra Guide

We will look at chakras in multiple ways throughout the book. The included tables focus on understanding the energetic meaning of thought and emotion that is associated with each chakra. Let's begin with the general function of chakras.

Each of the seven major chakras is positioned along the spinal column in a tornado-shaped funnel. Many people think that each chakra only spins outward through the front side of the body, but in fact, each chakra also forms a tornado-shaped funnel out the back of the body. At each chakra center, there are two spinning tornado forms, front and back, that seem to attach at the same point along the spine. The chakras seem to be the connection centers or points between the physical body, the spirit body, and the body of the universe.

Each chakra is an energy generator, carrying powerful energy signatures that correlate with significant life themes. Many people already realize that each chakra is represented by different colors. Each color the human eye sees registers as a certain frequency in our brain. Frequency is the number of times that a wave oscillates or repeats. The slower the wave oscillates, the darker the color and the denser the energy. The faster the wave oscillates, the lighter the color and the finer the energy. For instance, we see red at the base of a rainbow because it vibrates more slowly than orange, which is above it. The first chakra at the base of the spine vibrates in the denser red and the second chakra vibrates in the color of orange, etc.

Each chakra also generates an energy field inside and around the body. While some think each chakra creates an actual layer of energy around the body, it seems to be a more gradual intermingling of densities of energy, not defined layers around the body. Each organ and each joint also has minor chakra centers all intermingling with the major ones. The energy field of humans extends beyond the body and into the cosmos and at the same time extends down within the microcosm of each cell that makes up the physical body. The human body is not just muscle, bone, and brain. It is an alive, pulsating collection of energy.

The higher up the body each chakra is positioned, the less physically focused the energy is. As you learn to look into the chakras and the emerging energy, you will receive a general perspective of the major life themes and how that person is functioning or struggling with those life issues.

The human body is a smaller microcosm of the greater macrocosm, and the various energy centers of the body reflect major life themes within the realms of our development as conscious beings. Entering into the energy field is the first phase of entering into another person's intimate, personal story. For example, one would expect an energetically charged first and second chakra in a person who focuses on the physical world with its sexual or material pleasures, while a person such as Mother Teresa, who might have been focused more on the divine nature of the world, would have a more energetically charged sixth and seventh chakra.

As a person develops more love and understanding about self, the third chakra, also called the solar plexus, tends to appear in clear colors, vibrating in a higher range of energy. As that same person allows self-love, they begin to understand unconditional love, a love without criticism or judgment of others. As that person develops a purer love and understanding of people around them, the fourth chakra vibrates in a finer spectrum of greens and rose colors. As this person becomes more attuned to the divine will of Source, the fifth chakra energizes and expands in blues. This person lives more and more from the perspective that all is right within their body and mind.

When the sixth chakra, at the brow area, expands and hums in purple and violet shades, the person has advanced into a gentle ability of living from an insightful place. This perspective truly allows one to swim in an ocean of electrical energy that constantly provides intuitive information to live by. The road that was previously full of giant boulders is now a smoother road with an occasional bump of stone. This person senses life in vibrational, wave-like patterns of information and is aware of a higher intelligence guiding the way.

The seventh chakra links the physical human, living a physical life, with Divine Intelligence. This link is always there because each human is an active, vital factor in the whole story of the universe. When a person begins to live the life of a profoundly aware, unconditionally loving person, this energy center becomes a fountain of vital force energy rushing up into the heavens. The individual tends to respond to their physical life on earth rather than reacting to it. This person tends to be in a more constant prayerful state of being, aware of the interwoven matrix of the non-physical with the physical.

The chakras are displayed in a certain series of colors. Each color coincides with a general function. The functions of each chakra advance from the physical to the divine. Each chakra is just as important as another. Each center symbolizes profound aspects of the human condition and the development of each human as an individual. Please take note that most chakra charts and descriptions tend to show only the front of the body. Each chakra also has a corresponding spinning vortex along the back side of a person.

The colors of the major and minor centers will blend together or intermingle with a nearby chakra. The chakra centers are not isolated islands unto themselves. Energy at its finest is fluid, unbroken and even smooth as it emanates throughout the person.

The following two diagrams provide a quick view of the correlations between color, energy, emotions, and life awareness.

These diagrams provide a quick reference for the primary purpose and function of each chakra. You can utilize this information in the first sweep of someone's energetic field for an initial impression of their development and their struggles. After we discuss these general traits in the following paragraphs, you can then scan your own chakra centers in more depth.

Let's venture deeper and immerse ourselves in the chakras. There is more going on than we physical, breathing humans will ever know. For example, people who utilize the left brain in their life and their work, such as engineers, lawyers, or dentists, tend to have a very quiet, subdued seventh chakra. On the other hand, a nun, a daily meditator, or someone who frequently prays will have a surge of energy rising from the seventh. The energetic force from a chakra and also the direction of the flow will provide you with information imperative for a deeper understanding of your client's story.

We come into this life with a formulated energetic matrix or pattern that begins to shape who we are. This matrix expresses an electrical form for the human body. Each chakra generates and pulsates energy throughout the cells, organs, and tissues of the body. At the same time this rippling effect pulsates into the other chakras, creating other levels of a grid-like framework. As we mature, our thoughts, feelings, and choices reflect physically in the matrix and the chakras. Everything about this matrix interlinks to form the individual, and that same pulsating network joins a greater matrix, intertwining each of us into a unity of the whole.

The energy matrix of the lower chakras—the first, second, and third, for instance—contains a more condensed, compact wave frequency. While it is certainly not a rule, heavier emotions such as shame or guilt tend to resonate with the more physically based chakras and settle in, becoming thicker and resisting a healthy flow of energy, eventually manifesting as an illness or disease of some type. The remaining chakras also respond to positive or negative thought and emotion.

As you investigate the chakras, be aware of all the organs and body parts that lie within the area of each chakra. For instance, as you scan the heart chakra you can begin to sense that the lungs sit within that same area and are included within that energy center. Another example would be the third chakra. The energy of the solar plexus fans out from its centered point and includes the stomach, spleen, pancreas, gall bladder, liver, and even the kidneys. All of these organs reside nearby and are influenced primarily by that chakra but also a blend of adjacent chakras.

As you continue your medical intuition training you will naturally become more and more mindful of a finely tuned inter-connectedness of the human body, its organs, its systems, and its energy fields. You are entering into hidden levels of the individual's story. As a medical intuitive, you are assisting a person by discovering unrecognized concerns, issues, heartaches, and illness. People need our help at this level of healthcare.

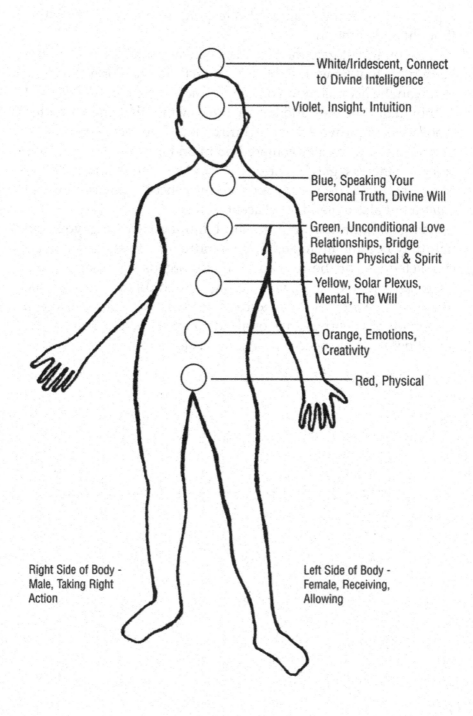

White/Iridescent, Connect to Divine Intelligence

Violet, Insight, Intuition

Blue, Speaking Your Personal Truth, Divine Will

Green, Unconditional Love Relationships, Bridge Between Physical & Spirit

Yellow, Solar Plexus, Mental, The Will

Orange, Emotions, Creativity

Red, Physical

Right Side of Body - Male, Taking Right Action

Left Side of Body - Female, Receiving, Allowing

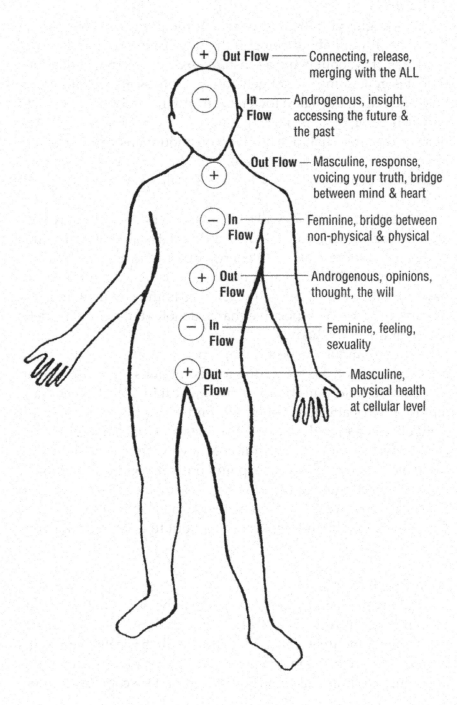

(+) Out Flow —— Connecting, release, merging with the ALL

(−) In Flow —— Androgenous, insight, accessing the future & the past

(+) Out Flow — Masculine, response, voicing your truth, bridge between mind & heart

(−) In Flow —— Feminine, bridge between non-physical & physical

(+) Out Flow — Androgenous, opinions, thought, the will

(−) In Flow —— Feminine, feeling, sexuality

(+) Out Flow — Masculine, physical health at cellular level

### First Chakra

Let's begin with the first chakra at the groin area and base of the spine. It is all about being in the physical world in a physical body. Yes, it is about being a sensual, sexual being, but at the same time it is generating, or not generating, a physical level of vitality. It is called the first chakra for a reason and that reason is the health and well-being of a functioning human body. Scanning the energy field of the first chakra will give you mountains of information about the general level of vigor, stamina, and liveliness of the individual before you. That liveliness will glow in clear, bright reds.

A healthy first chakra will feel and look vibrant, generally with an outward flowing force. Males and females alike will find this center has a more masculine energy due to the action of vitality and cellular health emanating outward. The first chakra is said to have a positive electrical charge. This has nothing to do with being a positive person. This positive charge denotes the electromagnetic aspect of the living body.

As one might suspect, many people suffer in the groin area and base of the spine due to sexual abuse and the human tendency to hold onto heavy emotions. I find that this chakra is almost always affected; rarely do I find it surging with energy. It symbolizes literally the base of all things material, all things of the earth, and the struggles we humans have with these issues. Like the roots of a tree, this center pours outward and down into the earth, connecting us to the physical, linking the physical body to the earth body. We are indeed one with the giant ball that we call our planet, and the first chakra reaches out to create that dynamic link.

### Second Chakra

The second energy center is below the belly button. In its healthy state it will frequently show itself in various shades of orange sometimes mingled with red. It basically represents creation. The male and female reproductive organs are in this area, but one must also consider the broader scope of creation.

This area symbolizes the ability of creating in one's own life. For example, one client recently yearned to be an artist but instead spent all of her time as an accountant because her parents valued that profession. Even though she always felt that the accounting profession was stifling, she did not follow her own guidance that told her she was an artist. Her second chakra reflected that repressed energy. In general, this area is about procreation and at the same time creating the individual we are meant to be. We are here to live our dreams and those dreams are coming from the voice of our soul. The second chakra is literally about being true to oneself.

This center is said to generate a negatively charged electromagnetic field. (This is not the same as negative emotions.) In both males and females, this chakra produces a more feminine energy, which would also denote a receptive feel. As you sense this center, notice if it feels like the flow of energy seems more incoming or outgoing. When all is well in this area of the body, the practitioner will sense an inflow of energy or the awareness of receiving. The stirring of creation through sexuality is there along with the stirring of our individual development.

### Third Chakra

This center is above the belly button and up toward the base of the rib cage. It is known as the solar plexus. It is about developing more and more as an individual. While it is a long distance from the brain, it is considered the center of our will, or the mental component. One might say, "How on earth does the upper abdomen relate to our mental abilities?" My short answer is that the mind is within every cell of who we are and the mind is equivalent to the energy of the soul. It is literally the core of who you are.

The solar plexus emanates with the individual's sense of self or the sense of our own individual empowerment. Individuality is more than just thought processes within the organ of the brain. When we are standing strong in our own empowerment, this area will look and feel like the bright yellow of sunshine on a cloudless day. Many people define the solar plexus as more androgynous, without male or female qualities. Standing strong with our values and feeling our personal sense of integrity is an aspect of females and males equally, making this center one of balance. This chakra should feel more outgoing than incoming. Its flow is outward, representing our place in the world as powerful creators.

### Fourth Chakra

Oh, the heart, the heart! The HeartMath Institute has not only discovered that the heart contains brain cells but it has also found that the heart retains memory like the brain. Have you read any accounts of people who have received heart transplants? After the transplant they often find that they now have new life interests and new food cravings. When researched they discover that the changes they are experiencing are identical to the lifestyle of the heart donor.

My friend's father received a heart transplant many years ago. When he went back to work he and his coworker found themselves lost in Indianapolis. Suddenly, my friend's father began directing the driver to turn this way and that way and they drove directly to their destination. This man had never been in Indianapolis before! Speculation says that the information came from the heart memory of the donor.

Over the years, I find myself telling clients that their breath is the bridge between the physical world and the non-physical world. The first thing we do at birth is take our first breath and breathe is the last thing that we do at the sacred passage of death. The lungs lie within the heart chakra and the two major organs, together, create a spirit bridge, uniting our physical nature with our soul essence.

While humanity already understands that the energy frequency of love comes from the heart center, humanity struggles with the concept that this love can be free flowing, without stipulations and without judgment or strings attached. True compassionate love, without any conditions attached to it and no matter what is said or done by others, is paramount for our higher expansion.

The heart center is primarily an intake center, and not an output center. Consider the significance of this for a moment. Could it be that the truth and power of this chakra is unconditional love for self, first and foremost? What would the ramifications of this concept be if we all began to apply it? When I bring this up to people, panic flashes across their faces. Then they immediately declare that they could never put themselves first because that is the foundation of selfishness.

Aren't we taught that we are to give and give to others without consideration of self?

Aren't we taught that focusing on self is selfish? Aren't we taught that life is painful and to toughen up? Aren't we taught love has strings attached?

Aren't we taught that we must work harder and provide materialistically for others?

Aren't we taught that people are only for themselves and you have to watch out?

These are the issues that I hear every day in my office from worn down and worn out people. These same people are afraid to be selfish. These same people have thick energetic protective barriers across their chests. Instead of allowing love to stream into their life and body, they keep pushing through life by doing and doing and doing for everyone except themselves. Because of this, these same people must create energetic protective barriers to help themselves get through it. The number of clients I have seen with protection covering their hearts is uncountable! If only each one of them only knew the more we care for and tend to ourselves first and foremost, the more we have to give. The more we have to give offers us the freedom of an open, unhidden heart.

Mark Nepo poetically describes the struggles within the human heart in *The Book of Awakening*: "Risk opens safety. It doesn't shut it down. Only through the risk to open can we inhabit and receive the strength and fullness of what is whole. This raises the very profound question of how to define self-protection. Is it hiding who you are or being who you are? Is it guarding yourself with all that you see or is it clearing yourself to let light in? Is it preparing yourself against all that can hurt you or is it opening yourself to all that can heal you?"

The heart chakra is an intake center. This is so important that I will repeat it. The heart chakra is an intake center. It is paramount that we receive and accept the finely tuned vibration of love into our being to energetically nourish our own body, mind, and soul. If you focus on receiving all that life has to offer, you will be empowered to give abundantly to others as a result. It is an intake center, not an output center. The heart center is the bridge between life's journey of the physical and life's journey of the soul. In health, the heart blends together greens of the physical world with pink, rich, rose colors of the spirit.

### Fifth Chakra

The throat is vulnerable. Struggles take place in life and are reflected in the neck and throat. The ability to express ourselves or to stifle that expression vibrates in this center. People often choose to stifle their truth for the sake of someone else. This chakra is about expressing the truth of what we think and feel from the depths of our soul outward to the world. The throat chakra will illustrate how the person handles their internal truth with the outside world. Do we communicate to the world or not?

Please note that communication is not exclusive to talking. There are myriad ways to express our individuality and our personal truth. One person might express their inner heart with song while another paints a picture on a public wall. There might be a song to sing or a blanket to crochet. One person may need to write a book and another will feel a deep satisfaction when they mimic a bird's song as they hike along a trail. The fifth chakra concerns the decisions to take right action or the decisions to not take right action in life. The focus of action signifies this center with male characteristics. Evidence of following one's soul direction will present itself in this chakra in blues and indigos.

This chakra vibrates as a bridge much like the heart chakra. The fifth chakra forms a vibrational link between the heart and the head. The function of a bridge is to offer equal passageway. In other words, this focal point within the neck and throat offers a balance within life between thinking and feeling. How often have you found yourself making statements such as "She is totally in her head all the time" or "He is all heart." The general public, who are usually not consciously aware of energy, make these types of comments all the time. Little do they know that they are accurately describing what the medical intuitive is deeply aware of.

### Sixth Chakra
Here is the seat of the third eye. What does that truly mean? The portrayal of this center as an eyeball probably originated due to its function of seeing without actual, physical eyeballs. This center has the capacity to consciously perceive non-physical awareness with the greater soul-self. Here is the ability to perceive the non-physical realm with compassionate understanding of the earth realm. This chakra vibrates at its finest when the individual advances into true insight with compassionate understanding of the world and its multifaceted cultures and individuals. Utilizing our intuitive guidance diminishes criticism and judgment and unlocks the fascinated observer within to perceive all creation as exquisite. While some people describe this chakra in blues, I personally perceive and feel it to have the frequency of purples.

Many people struggle to enhance their innate intuitive abilities. Clients tell me that they spend a great deal of time sending energy out through the third eye in an attempt to become clairvoyant, only to find their perceptions do not improve. It is important to note that this chakra is an intake center, not an output center. Perceiving is a passive activity. It is a matter of noticing and receiving the information that people and nature provide for us every moment of our waking and sleeping life. This is a receptive chakra. The fascinated observer does not jump into the action. Rather, in a state of great wisdom, they observe, detect, and take note of the countless ways that understanding and intelligence reside universally.

### Seventh Chakra

I do not usually visualize this chakra in white but I see it as shimmering iridescence of all colors. Remember blowing bubbles outdoors and watching the sun shine through them? It is a combination of all visible colors and yet it is transparent. Its clarity seems to float in the breeze of energy. We are not separate from the grander whole of it all. Each human is a portion or segment of all that is. We are tapped into the totality whether we are aware of it or not. Selecting to tap in with clear, conscious awareness, in my humble opinion, is where the rubber meets the road. The more we consciously connect our body, our emotions, and our thoughts, the more we stand as creators of life.

You might notice in the future that many of your clients have diminished energy in the crown center. If it is difficult to feel or see energy at the top of your client's head, you can understand that this person does not pray or meditate or give much consideration to the spiritual aspect of their life. I can confidently tell you that people who do not have activated crown chakras will describe greater struggles and conflicts in their lives than people who have energy flowing in the seventh chakra. Anyone who prays, meditates, or gives some consideration to their spiritual life will have quite a force rushing upward. I have actually been blown backwards by the force from one man's crown chakra. This man had spent a great deal of his life in deep meditation.

The seventh center, at the crown of who we are, emanates with an outward current just like the first chakra. Consider this. Each human being is an interweaving vessel of energy that contacts the earth through the first chakra, and at the same time bonds us to the entire galaxy and beyond. A soul in a human body has the ability and choice to become one with the physical and at the same time one with the Universe. We hold a vital position as a conduit for the empowered force of the universe. People—yes, you and me—have a divine importance in the creation and the development of the All.

Now I ask you to slow down. For just a few moments, do an internal scan of your seven major chakras. Decide to be a fascinated observer of your own body. You may begin at the top of your head and move downward or begin in your groin area and sweep upward. It might seem as if you are walking around down inside of your own body.

As before, write down your immediate impressions as you scan yourself. Document each one in your journal as it happens. Do not censor it in any way. Write down absolutely everything, even if it seems inconsequential. Do not ignore any details that suddenly rise up as if out of nowhere. If you find yourself ignoring a piece of information that pops in, you might realize that is exactly the issue you are struggling with. It is time to check it out and learn about you. Don't worry or be afraid. Deep down you already know it anyway, but now it is time to know and understand yourself at a more significant level.

## Steps for Your Inner Chakra Awareness

1.  Prepare yourself to notice anything and everything that pops up. Notice the most instant information that comes up and do not discard anything.

2.  Send yourself into a quiet, meditative place.

3.  Begin at either your head or the base of your spine. It is your decision where to begin.

4.  Send your fascinated observer right into the energy center. Your mind will feel itself focusing on that area. Take note that each chakra emanates through the front of your body and also note the backside of each chakra along the spine.

5.  Notice the feel of each chakra—alive, sleepy, stagnant, flowing, or something else.

6.  Notice the look of the area—color, darkness, brightness, images, symbols.

7. Notice the movement—the direction of movement or the lack of movement.

8. Notice the size and shape of the chakra. Are some larger or smaller than the others?

9. Notice any emotions or feelings, any aches or pains, in each area.

10. Ask each chakra to tell you something about it. Take the first word or phrase that pops into your mind.

Describe your insights in your journal now. Repeat this inner self-discovery frequently.

# Chapter Eight

## Prepare for Body Awareness

### Know the Body in a Different Way

You do not need a medical background to offer a medical intuitive session. You do need to know the basics about the human body, including where all the organs and body parts are generally located and especially how that organ or area of the body responds to our thoughts and emotions.

So far, we have discussed the aura as a living force field that courses throughout the body and projects outward beyond the skin. We reviewed the major chakra system with the implications and meaning for each energy center and how it correlates with the environment around us. Now, in a very easy to understand way, we need to review the internal organs, where they are located, their function within the body, and their correlation to illness, disease, and well-being.

Energetically, the body as a whole represents two activities: receiving and giving. Whether we are male or female in our current body, we naturally have male and female characteristics. Even a male who has strong male characteristics might exhibit issues or conflicts regarding female traits. In the same manner, you might find yourself scanning an extremely feminine woman only to find an area of disease concerning male-like qualities. No matter how they appear or interact in life, a male body integrates both male and female qualities and the female body integrates both male and female qualities.

The right side of our body signifies the more male quality of taking action or not taking action. It involves taking steps in life and following through, or its opposite, the inability to take action. The right side of the body also embodies male type themes in life such as:

- Taking care of self.
- Feeling confident, energized, and powerful.
- Taking care of others.
- Awareness of creating goals.
- Taking the correct steps in life to achieve one's goals.
- Standing strong in one's values when others disagree.
- Outwardly expressing self and being seen out in the world.
- Choosing the right job for one's values.
- Taking a hike in the mountains because one feels alive in the mountains.

Please note that struggles on the right half of the body may also denote struggles with males in life. The influencing male could be anyone: a neighbor, a brother, uncle or father, a son, a boss, or a school teacher. Illness usually develops or presents itself physically when someone ruminates about that male or the situation regarding that male. Going over and over something in our mind will give the issue more physical substance, resulting in a physical disorder.

Remember, the more we repeatedly think and feel something, the more compact or solid the energy becomes, either positively or negatively. The repetition of thought and emotion creates a more physical and complex outcome in the body. If the focus is on the positive, then the body responds to that positive energy, but if the ruminating is more negative in nature, the body will suffer the outcome of negativity. When a more masculine trait presides, the body will often display some type of struggle on the right side or right half of the person.

The female qualities pertain generally to the left half of the human body. The left side of the body, whether male or female, characterizes female qualities. Like the male side, the female side of the body concerns female life qualities but also the females in one's family or social circle. Like the males, these females could be a mother, aunt, a teacher, boss, or any relationship with a significant female.

It is a female characteristic to be a receptacle with the ability or the inability to receive in life. Female themes portrayed in life will include but are certainly not limited to such things as:

- Being able to rest or even take a nap.
- Accepting gifts.
- Graciously accepting positive comments from others.
- Nurturing others.
- Allowing oneself to be nurtured.
- Receiving financial payment based on your true sense of worth.
- Receiving other types of reimbursement for one's efforts.
- Receiving the sweetness of life.
- The ability to stop activity.
- Noticing and allowing one's intuition.

Receiving in one's life is often a dramatic struggle between fears of becoming selfish or the joy of becoming selfless. Many cultural standards tend to create expectations that limit the evolution of the individual for the sake of the society. These limitations often begin the creation of physical struggles that lead to physical illness. When I listen to my clients I often hear questions such as "Is it all right to receive?" or "What should I receive in my life?" and "How much can I receive and how much is too much?" Do you hear the emotional struggle beneath those questions? I hear thoughts and emotions of shame, guilt, and self-deprivation. Take this opportunity to teach that the Universe is abundant and ready to give richly if we choose to receive. It is a choice.

Male and female qualities also have physical traits that appear in the human brain. WebMD.com describes the two sides or hemispheres of the brain in the following way: "The two different sides or hemispheres are responsible for different types of thinking. Most individuals have a distinct preference for one of these styles of thinking and tend to have one side of the brain function much more than the other. For example, left hemisphere thinkers are logical, analytical, objective, while right hemisphere thinkers are intuitive, creative, subjective, holistic thinkers."

The medical field understands that the hemispheres of the human brain function in contrasting modes, and we humans tend to excel more strongly in one hemisphere while functioning less in the opposite hemisphere. For example, an engineer or a scientist might display more left brain traits because their focus in life is detail and logic based. Their work and their innate interests create an enhancement of electrical charges throughout the left brain. On the other hand, a professional medium or an artist would quite naturally have a more prominent right hemisphere, which functions in conceptual thinking and intuition.

Notice that the right and left brain function seem to be the opposite of the right and left energetic qualities in the rest of the human body. In other words, I discussed that the left half of the body tends to have female traits while the right half displays male aspects. Notice that the brain's functional traits seem to be in the reverse. You might remember in school that you were taught that vision from the right eye crosses over to the left side of the brain for processing and the nerves from the left eye transfer to the right side of the brain.

As a result, the female characteristics and also female struggles tend to present themselves physically on the left side of the body but cross over to the right side of the brain. The male characteristics and struggles tend to appear in the right side of the body but are distinguished as a left brain function.

Your next step is to understand the deeper concepts and meaning within the tissues and organs of an individual. Do not waste years of your medical intuitive work like I have. Get the impact of the following concept right now because here is the juice of it:

**Essential Point:**
*Each thought and each emotion that a human thinks*
*and feels connects directly with a specific organ*
*or area of the body or system of the body.*

To clarify that statement, I will give you some simple examples. The shoulders of the human body are structured to carry loads. When we carry something heavy, we tend to carry it on our shoulders because of the strength of the muscles in that area of the body. The man who brings salt to my house for the water softener carries the bags on his shoulders. Shoulders are structured to carry physical loads but also tend to carry energetic burdens.

Let's continue to give more definition to this example. When you assess the individual and discover the energy of the left shoulder seems heavy and thick, you may be picking up certain struggles this person is having. This person may be taking on too many tasks or responsibilities and it is weighing them down. Remember, the left side of the body is about positively receiving or the more negative trait of taking on more than one can handle.

If the right shoulder looks or feels thick and heavy, you might understand that the person is struggling or confused about taking too much action regarding the burdens they are carrying. They find themselves physically running around each day taking care of everyone's needs. As an example, this person will be doing everything for their children but also their neighbors, and at the same time they are volunteering at two different organizations, etc. In other words, they simply cannot ever say no to anyone.

Let's look at that same example on the positive end of the spectrum. Let's say that your scan picks up that one shoulder or even both look healthy. The energetic colors and the feel of the shoulders is clear, smooth, and flowing. You can inform your client that they are not taking on too much and they are doing well with the responsibilities in their life.

When I asked the man who delivers my salt about his shoulders, he said the weight does not bother him. His response alone tells me that he is balanced in life regarding responsibilities because those bags of salt that he carries all day long do not bother him.

Let's discuss another example of how the right and left side of the body give us more information concerning the mind, the emotion, and the body relationship. I had a horrible, sharp pain radiating throughout the left side of my buttocks for a long period of time. I finally stopped and asked myself about the pain in my butt and up popped my mother. Aha! My mother issues were in my butt! Let's look at this example in a medically intuitive manner. What are hips and the buttocks about? If you say that the hips are about balance and structure of the body, you are correct. To understand this even more specifically, our buttocks literally represent that which we sit on. The entire back side of the human body represents what is behind us in our past.

Let's make the connections between emotions, thoughts, and our physical body. Most of my issues with my mother were coming from our past together when I was a child. Rather than looking at a particular issue with conscious awareness, I began to sit on the pain of my past rather than looking at it. My emotional pain was sharp and knife-like, and so was my physical pain. It was manifesting in the hip area because I was dealing with the basic structure of my life with all of its ups and downs. It was specifically on the left side of my hips because I was taking on a great deal of responsibility for my mother as she reached the later years of her life.

Is this all beginning to come together for you? My examples of the water softener man and my hips are the types of everyday issues you will find as a medical intuitive. It is imperative, however, to learn and incorporate this extremely natural connection between mind, emotions, and our body. Set your intent now to formulate these natural relationships between thought, feeling, and the physical body. Become conscious of this relationship and you will spontaneously open the current of instinctive intuition.

Watch and listen to normal, everyday comments. People have naturally coined terms such as:

"He is a pain in my neck."

"I just can't swallow this any longer."

"She was a pain in my butt."

"I feel like I am shouldering the weight of the world."

"He acts like he is carrying the weight of the world on his back."

People are unconsciously describing the bodymind connection in these comments. Be careful not to make this type of comment about your own life. That which repeats in our minds and emotions will have more substance, more volume, and become more solid. Remember that thoughts and emotions, positive or negative, are energetic substances floating throughout our cells, our tissues, our organs, and our bones. Take charge of your thoughts and emotions, and you will naturally take charge of your body.

### Essential Point:
*Take charge of your thoughts and emotions and you will naturally take charge of your body.*

### Our Current Life Affects Our Current Body

My sister and I sometimes discuss our painful and abusive upbringing. We have also discussed how it has affected our emotional bodies and our physical bodies. In my more recent lectures, I discuss the fact that the happier I get, the more easily I have been able to release the burdens of painful emotions.

My sister has multiple sclerosis, which creates a scarring within the brain and along the length of the nerves. My sister tells me that I have spent thousands of dollars in therapy regarding our childhood (which I agree), while she has done her best to never look into her personal past again.

Each of us can certainly understand my sister's unwillingness and refusal to think about or process her pain and anger. Her continued refusal over the years may have enhanced the disease process, however. The underlying issue beneath multiple sclerosis is about communication. The brain and nervous system constantly receive emotional signals saying, "Stop thinking, remembering, or feeling." Those emotional "thought signals" carry messages to the physical body, and the body must respond to that energy. In this case, multiple sclerosis complies and my sister's brain and nervous system create scar tissue. The scars thicken and the thoughts and emotions slow down. Can you see the natural fit between the two?

On a positive note, my sister has the survival instincts of a fighting rooster. I think she is amazing in all that she does and accomplishes from a wheelchair!

If you think this is all an oversimplification of life, I agree with you. There is certainly more going on than we mere humans can conceive of. Many people ask, "What about children that come into the world already sick or the ones who die soon after birth? Are you saying they are to blame for their illness?"

Illness and disease are never about blame. They are, however, signals from our thoughts and subsequent emotions. These signals can give us all types of information and opportunities to learn and understand the world within and the world without.

No one is to blame. We are never to succumb to blame no matter the age of the individual. The energetic vibration of blame is squelching, heavy, and suffocating. Blaming others and blaming ourselves creates a dramatic kink in our energy field, preventing the intelligence of a situation to come through. Every experience, every situation, is another layer of learning and another opportunity to expand our soul's development.

The illness may have its origins from an individual's ancestry or even from a past life. It is also never about punishment. Everything in this life is a continuum of all that is and all that we are and have been. Each experience, even illness, offers an opportunity to learn a deeper level of awareness. Punishment is a concept created by humans, not by Source. We live in a magnificently complicated system of experiences. Our current experiences are interwoven within our past lives and our future possibilities. Through this lacing of experiences and repetitive themes, our life generates new situations to learn and expand from.

Our body speaks to us. It is a dynamic part of the whole experience of learning. It speaks to us when we are deep within a state of well-being. It speaks to us when we have a cold and it speaks to us when we succumb to a terminal illness. The human body and personality are not to be blamed but to be understood.

The body is an intricate portion of our entire experience, but it is only a portion. The people that you assist with medical intuition will often blame themselves or God or someone else. Assist them to sense the total story of their life and not just the disease. Our human body is only participating with the grander story for each of us.

**Essential Point:**
*Humans tend to blame others, but our struggles only reflect what we are trying to learn.*

I am convinced that the mind and soul are one and the same. The mind is not only located in the brain but it resides within every cell and tissue of the body. The mind/soul is not contained within the boundaries of the skin. It dwells within the body and beyond the body. The mind/soul weaves within each cell of the body and at the same time it interweaves within the cosmos. The living human is a participant in the world and a participant with Source.

## Relationships Affect Our Health

One of the most impactful influences in our life and in our physical body is our relationships. Relationships include everyone that you come in contact with. Relationships may include the clerk at the drug store or the conductor in the subway. I now have a relationship with the contractor who built my beautiful screened-in porch and the man who took the potholes out of my driveway. The telemarketer who called you on the phone last night at dinnertime connected with you in some level of relationship.

During her medical intuitive session with me, Lynn revealed through her energy the effect of an unhealthy relationship. I told her, "I see a deep tunneling of dark maroon energy going right down into your heart. This tunneling is something literally eating away at you. There seems to be almost nothing left of you in this situation with someone. I am actually quite concerned for you at this time. Not only is there little energy within the organ of your heart, there is this empty tunnel, which should not be there. It has not taken over your heart completely because I can still see some of the heart muscle, but the tunnel consumes much of it."

I went on to say in a soft, compassionate voice, "Nothing is coming into your heart center to replenish it. You simply do not know how to replenish it at this point." Lynn interrupted me to state in a sad, quiet voice that she was the only caretaker for her elderly mother. She had been the caretaker for her mother for years and struggled with the responsibilities.

I asked Lynn to give me only the first name of her mother, which she did without hesitation. The moment Lynn verbalized her mother's name, a hand instantly rose up and came at me, trying to stab me in the heart!

Let's stop here for a moment and discuss this situation. While this experience surprised me, I was not fearful, nor did it injure me in anyway. This did not physically happen to me nor did I take that negative energy into my own body. I did not even receive the energy of being stabbed in the heart. I experienced a message about Lynn's mother—a powerful message.

This is very important for the new medical intuition student to understand and come to terms with. I witnessed intuitive information about the relationship between Lynn and her mother. This symbol and the action of this symbol said it all. I received a message about the energetic action of this mother toward her daughter, and I also received a message about the energetic consequences for Lynn. The tunnel was eating away at her heart, her body, and her aura. Lynn constantly felt hostility from her mother and tearfully said it was like a knife in her heart every day.

Lynn explained that her mother was extremely critical and

harshly lashed out, belittling Lynn on a daily basis. I watched her energy as she talked and cried. I saw a baby glowing in golden light. "I see that you have been working on healing since you were first born," I said to her softly. She told me that at birth the cord was wrapped around her neck, and she was about to be pronounced dead, but when the cord was removed she began to breathe.

We can learn so much from relationships. Each interactive relationship is rich with opportunity to learn about ourselves while we learn about another. What many people fail to consider is that each person has 50 percent of the responsibility of what happens in a relationship, even in the case of Lynn and her hostile mother. Lynn's participation with her mother and the manner in which she participated was 50 percent of what happened.

The relationship was taking its toll on Lynn. She had a huge variety of choices that would shift the energetic drain and the empty tunneling in her heart. If she chose not to change, she may receive a more severe diagnosis from her doctor than what she had at this point.

A few days later I was deep into a different reading with a different person. I could feel this person had made huge decisions lately. "I see a man with black hair who looks like an Aztec. He has dark skin, black hair, and deep, dark eyes. He is right up in my face, but now he turns his head and looks back over his left shoulder. He is looking at you way back in his past. When I follow his gaze, I see you very bright with light all around you. He knows that you are healing and making transformations that are positive for you. He feels heavy and sad that he is so far from you."

My client told me, "I am going through a divorce right now and he is Mexican. Your description of him and what is going on is accurate. I had to make this change for me." I told her that the changes are already very positive for her and reminded her that I see her literally glowing because of it. This woman made a choice to take care of herself and was allowing her ex-husband to take responsibility for himself. The more we attempt to carry the responsibility of others, the more burdened we will become.

Our lifestyle, the choices and the decisions that we make, have an effect on our bodies. Our heads are indeed connected to our bodies. The bodymind unit, as mentioned earlier and as coined by Candace Pert in *Molecules of Emotion,* experiences every positive and every negative occurrence right along with you. What happens inside of us is a reflection of what we think and feel about the life around us. The happier we consistently become emotionally, the happier our bodies become. It is said that love makes the world go round.

I have a healing story to illustrate the vibration of love. My dear friend Louise received the diagnosis of uterine cancer, stage three. Frightened and alarmed, she called me. I asked her to come to my office so I could have a look into her energy field and her body. We met soon after the call and both settled into a meditative state.

I sent my energy toward her as she sat across from me. Rather than doing a full scan from the head down, I focused on the problem area. I saw a million or more black dots the size of pin points floating in her lower abdomen. The dots formed a dark hazy cloud centered in the second chakra area. I told her that I do not usually see cancer so diffuse, that for me there was usually a black shiny solid form. As I stated the words to her a wave of calm washed over me and I felt very positive about her condition.

When I reported what I saw and felt, Louise reminded me that the cancer was diagnosed as stage three and that stage four is the worst. I told her that I knew it was a severe diagnosis but energetically it still had not formed and organized itself and that seemed quite positive to me. I told her that I had some "homework" for her to do but it was totally up to her if she did it.

My guides directed me to ask Louise to practice her homework with me as we sat in my office. I asked her to place her own hands on her lower abdomen, right over the location of the uterus. I then asked her to remember the feeling of being overcome with a physical sensation of deep love. The physical sensation of love is different for each one of us. That moment of love might feel like your heart swells to its bursting point or it might feel like a warm wave of water flooding over you with fullness and warmth or it might be something else to you.

Louise said she had felt that in the past and knew what I meant. She became quiet and recreated that physical response inside of herself. I asked her to send it flowing down her arms and into her uterus. Even the air in the room changed as she did this. It felt lighter and easier to breathe as we continued on in quiet. I gave Louise this particular homework because it jumped into my mind as if from out of nowhere. I then received information that she was to send that vibration of love into that area three times a day until the surgery.

Bless her heart. Louise did her homework for the three weeks prior to the scheduled surgery. When she went back for her post-surgery checkup, the doctor told her that they were surprised to find that the cancer was not as developed and not as large as the scan had shown. What they removed was considered stage two. The doctor would probably deny that the "homework" had any effect on the cancer.

Others would say that was a coincidence. I say there are no coincidences. We can be divinely guided by receiving organized information from Spirit or we can ignore it and struggle alone. It's our choice.

**Human Anatomy Simplified**

You do not need to take an anatomy course and memorize the human anatomy. You do need to have some basic awareness, and you can do it with the help of the simplified diagram on the next page. The hardest part of this is to make sure you are aware that the right and left side of your client's body as you sit in front of them is not the same as your right and left side. Sometimes I have to stop and make sure that I am accurate about the side of their body I am referring to because the person sitting before you is facing you—their right side is really to your left and vice versa.

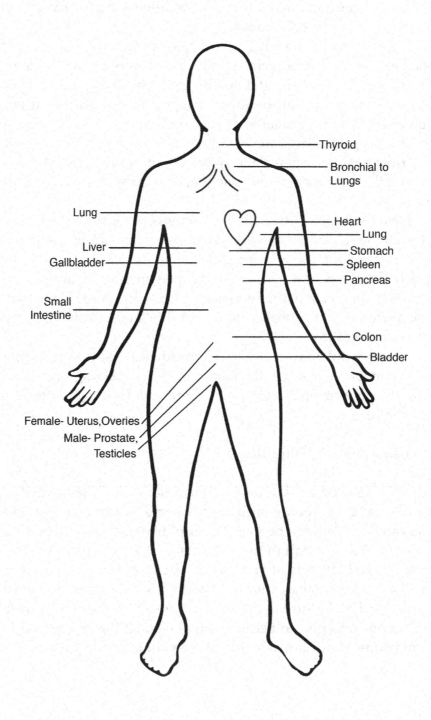

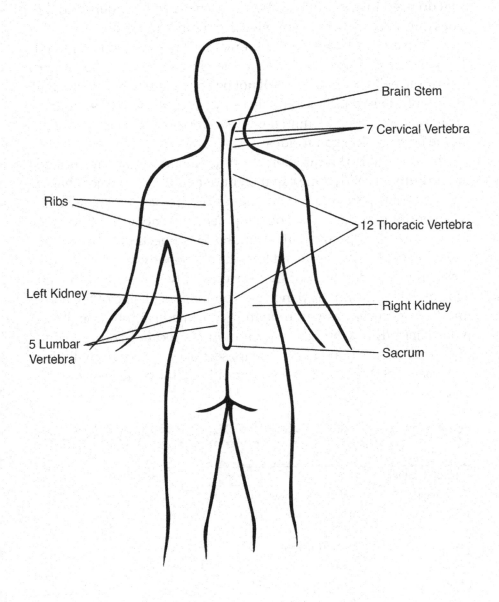

The two diagrams of the human body show a front view and a back view. While you do not really need a class in anatomy nor do you really need to know what each organ looks like anatomically, you do need to know the location of each organ to understand the bodymind connection as you visualize with x-ray eyes.

For example, if you do not know that the stomach is centered high in the abdomen just below the rib cage and is not down below the belly button, you will not be able to describe a particular illness of the stomach accurately. As you learn the following two diagrams, also keep in mind the importance of knowing what side of the body each organ resides.

It is essential to know where the fundamental organs are located in the human's body. One can then understand what major chakra oversees each particular organ that resides in that general area. As you continue through your development as a medical intuitive, it is also important to make the mindbody connection between the meaning behind the right and left side of the body. In other words, knowing that the organ of the heart actually sits over to the left side of the body and the pancreas is on the far left side of the body may be significant as you tune into your medical intuition about your client. Knowing where each organ is located and knowing the primary function of each organ, section, and system will give you reams of information as you intuitively move deeper into the body.

| Mind-Emotion-Body Connections Table | | |
|---|---|---|
| Body Part | Physical Function | Struggle with |
| Head/Shoulders | | |
| Left Brain | Analyzing, details, logic | Clear thinking, avoid feeling |
| Right Brain | Imagination, creativity, concepts | Creativity, imagination |
| Face | Structure of identity | Own identity, being seen |
| Sinus | Open areas of nasal system | Annoyed, tears not cried |
| Eyes | Sight of physical world | See the world as it really is |
| Ears | Sound of physical world | Hear the world as it really is |
| Jaw/Teeth | Speech/eating | Ruminating, receiving |

| | | |
|---|---|---|
| Throat/Neck | Connecting head with body | Express individual truth, swallow someone else's truth |
| Thyroid | Metabolism, growth | Secrets, limitations, abilities |
| Shoulders/arms/hands | Action | Too much action, responsibilities, I am the only one |
| **Chest** | | |
| Bronchial Tubes | Pathway to lungs | Restricted, arguments, stuck |
| Lung | Collection/distribution of air | Unable to live own rhythm/cycle, excessive sadness, grief |
| Heart | Pump for circulation | Not flowing in life, no joy, hardened emotions |
| Breast | Supply milk | Worthiness, everyone more important than self, self-nourishment, mothering issues |
| Rib cage | Protects heart/lungs | Vulnerable, victim, no protection |
| **Upper Abdomen** | | |
| Stomach | Collects/digests | Irritation, self-worth, nourish others to own detriment, who is the real me |
| Gallbladder | Creates bile, digests fats | Holding onto heavy emotions, hardened emotions, bitterness |
| Liver | Digests, metabolizes toxins | Not processing strong emotions, rage, toxic emotions |
| Spleen | Filters, recycles, fights bacteria | No life flow, overwhelmed |
| Pancreas | Produces insulin and digestive enzymes | Relying on external sources for the good things in life, life did not become sweet like I thought it would |
| **Lower Abdomen** | | |
| Colon | Holds waste | Stagnation, unable to process life events, holding onto old memories and old pain |
| Intestines | Absorbs nutrients | Unable to understand real life, life does not give to me |
| Ovaries | Holds eggs, produces hormones | Unable to create life for self and others |
| Uterus | Holds fetus | Home as a child or adult, form own life |
| Prostate | Nourishes/protects sperm | Struggle to protect and survive, pressured by life, giving up |

| Testicles | Creates sperm | Did not create the life I wanted |
|---|---|---|
| Hips | Skeletal form connecting trunk and legs | Little or no foundation for self |
| **Legs** | | |
| Knees | Joint for movement of legs | Obstinacy, inflexible, rigid in life |
| Ankles | Joint for movement of feet | Tension, hardened about flow of life |
| Feet | Structure to stand/move | Not grounded, fear of life changes and moving forward |
| **Back** | | |
| Spine | Supports body, protects spinal column | Wants more support, more communication, victim, powerless |
| Kidneys | Filters blood, controls fluid | Blames self/others, negative, criticism, disappointment |
| Adrenal glands | Create hormones to handle stress | It's all too much, no self-care |
| Buttocks | Muscles supporting back | The past, sitting on unresolved past and old pain |
| **Body Systems** | | |
| Lymph | Immune system, flow of body fluid, kills bacteria | Unable to defend self, flow with life |
| Blood vessels | Distribution of blood | Pathways of life, making connections, movement |
| Bones/muscles | Form structure of body | Strength, support, structure in life |
| Skin | Organ covering body | What world sees, protection of self |
| Nerves | Pathway between brain and body | Interconnections, communication breakdown |

It is crucial to understand the inherent relationship between the biology of the human body and the energy of thought and emotion. When you understand the most basic function and purpose of a body part, you can understand the very basic energy of thought that tends to settle within that body part. Like does attract like. Continuous repetitive thoughts and their subsequent emotions will tend to settle within the body part whose role is similar to the topic of that thought.

# Chapter Nine

## Prepare for the Unusual and the Not So Unusual

**Past Lives and Our Current Body**

"I do not know how else to tell you this except to describe it to you," I said to Linda, my client on the other end of the phone. "As I project toward you, I keep seeing your head floating up and away from your body and then it returns for a moment and then it lifts away again. Your head appears in dense red and black and dark, thick purple as it floats above your body. Thoughts separate from your body and you are very angry. It continues to drift over to your left."

I described this to her in my calm, professional medical intuitive voice. "I am sensing a traumatic past life for you. Oh . . . now I instantly see a sword swinging through your neck and now your head has fallen and is rolling across a wooden platform. Now the head rolls over the edge of the platform and falls to the ground.

"Your entire body looks open and empty like a grave. Your energy shows anger in dark maroon red." I went on to tell her that her stomach was clenched with high anxiety and in the upper right quadrant there was an ulcerated, raw-looking area. Linda confirmed that she has a lot of pain in that exact spot. She said that complementary healthcare practitioners keep telling her that her adrenals are shot. Since she interjected with that information, I specifically looked at the top of her kidney area where the adrenals sit and saw that they were dim and depleted.

I told Linda she must first identify how enraged she was. Rage was draining her. We discussed issues about identifying her truth and the individual that she truly is. Please note that the human core, that which identifies us as an individual, sits literally within the core of our body where the solar plexus resides. Anatomically, the organ of the stomach also resides in this area, thus the stomach problems. Linda's current body displayed a red-hot thyroid where her past body was sliced in two. The throat area is about the outward expression of self. I went on to inform her that in this past life, her spirit hovered around for a long time after decapitation. It seems as if the horror of the situation had returned within her current life. As a result, Linda stated that she was terrified to be who she really was and to express who she really was. She concluded for herself that if she let anyone know her true thoughts she would probably die.

I am serious when I say that this strange past life information made complete sense to my client. Linda began to describe the pain and difficulties with her neck and shoulders in her current life. I told her that she also seemed to struggle with mental challenges such as organization of thoughts and her memory, sometimes feeling muddled even when she was not tired.

"Yes!" she exclaimed, "You are so right! I feel like I struggle with my head all the time." She also confirmed that the emotion of fear always seemed to lock into her throat and the muscles of her neck.

As a past life and life between lives regression facilitator, I must say that nothing surprises me anymore. People's experiences are astounding, intimate, blessedly sacred, and sometimes a great surprise. I have found that my training as a mental health counselor and hypnotherapist, as well as a professional intuitive medium, prepared me for the entire continuum of the human experience, past, present, and future. I absolutely know that my life and the lives of others continue on and on and on. How could we not be influenced by that continuum?

**Essential Point:**
*People's experiences are astounding, intimate,*
*blessedly sacred, and sometimes a great surprise.*
*Stop thinking of them as a punishment.*

While in my current body living on this earth, I have personally merged into the spirit realm and experienced segments of my life in the non-physical. I have also sat in awe with thousands of clients as they entered into their own spiritual experiences in the non-physical realm. I have held in-depth conversations with people in spirit and have continually received evidence that the information they reveal is accurate. I know with every cell of my being that this life is only a miniscule portion of a massive, intricate continuum.

A quote from Gary Schwartz in *The Living Energy Universe* speaks to this continuum: "Could it be that the pulsing vibrations that reverberate and remember throughout the evolving universe reflect the essence of the heart of the cosmos, the gift of loving energy to us all? Is the heart of the universe universal living memory? Our logical brains have been trained to say, 'It can't be so.' Our hearts simply say, 'I hope so.'"

Jane called from another state for her reading. I began the session. "A very dark form has recently lifted from your head area. You have released a very old negative way of thinking."

Jane became excited and exclaimed, "I have absolutely stopped trying to make my miserable husband happy!"

I giggled with her and went on to say, "Well, the anger is now outside of your head. It is still hovering nearby, but it is not coming from inside of you in this moment. You are releasing very old, old issues regarding anger."

Jane replied, "I no longer get angry at him. He is who he is and there is nothing that I can do that will change that."

I left Jane's head and continued to scan her neck, head, and chest. "There is a shield over your heart and you are wearing it like a piece of clothing. Oh, now I see. Jane, it appears like a bulletproof vest." I told her that she was prepared for an attack and that her attacks came like verbal bullets from others. She told me about a very long, tumultuous relationship with her daughter as well as her husband.

"Your solar plexus is newly bright with orange and yellows. I can tell this by the light shade of these colors, and they have not had time to develop into richer hues. I can see that you are truly feeling more of your own empowerment." Jane agreed that after she altered her thoughts about her husband she has felt a new lease on life.

I continued my assessment and found that Jane's hips were not in alignment. One hip appeared higher than the other. "Your hips are off balance. Our hips are about the balance of life. They are reflective of security in all types of ways," I continued. Jane replied that she always felt off balance and gave me some examples.

I felt like things were going quite well for this reading as I continued the scan but the second I assessed her legs, ankles, and feet, I saw an antique looking ball and chain around Jane's left ankle. Suddenly a young, thin, black male was looking at me. He immediately turned away and ran as fast as he could possibly go. I saw him running away many, many times only to be hauled back by his white male owner. I was sitting with this white, upper middle-class woman in her sixties but was seeing her past life as a teenage Afro-American male slave.

The images and the young man's emotions had taken over. I continued to watch as a neutral observer, like watching an old movie. When the owner had enough of chasing down his property, he hammered a metal cuff in place around the young slave's left ankle. A chain and heavy ball extended from the cuff. The iron was never removed and the young man grew into a full-sized man. As he grew, the cuff dug deeper into his ankle. The slave owner did not care at all about the damage it was doing. As the boy's body grew, the rusting cuff embedded into the man's leg permanently.

"My husband was my owner! Wasn't he, Tina?" Jane said in tears.

"It seems like it," I responded, "but you are the only one who knows for sure." She told me about being a slave to her husband and his needs. She had tried for over forty years to please him or help him or make him happy. She went on to say that she had always enjoyed being around Afro-American people and especially loved the openness of black women in their culture.

Take note: Jane also informed me that she'd had multiple surgeries on that ankle over the past years and actually had metal plates embedded in her ankle. Was I sensing the metal of her slave life and also the metal in the ankle of her current body? Even more important, as I continued to see Jane for counseling and she began to heal emotionally, she had the metal plates removed from her ankle!

This is worth repeating. As this woman healed emotionally, something changed in her ankle and eventually the surgeon removed the metal plates that bound her even in this life. My only part in it was envisioning the past life connection and informing my client about it. I did not interpret it for her. She already knew the connection and experienced an "aha" moment. The old chains snapped from her history, from her energy and, as a result of all of her work, from her body. This woman now appears brighter and brighter every time I see her.

Angie's case also describes an example of a past life trauma continuing to affect a person in their current life. Angie did not schedule a past life regression. She, in fact, came to me for what I call "regular" or traditional hypnosis for migraines. While I have specialized as a regressionist, I also see many clients for life issues such as phobias, pain, excellence in sports, and a wide variety of other concerns. Angie, now in her late forties, came from a fundamental Christian upbringing and she had continued a conservative lifestyle throughout her adult life.

As she entered my office, Angie was quite anxious and somewhat fearful about hypnosis but was desperate to get relief from migraine pain. I did my best to relieve her anxiety as I described what clinical hypnosis really is. She agreed to continue with the session and stretched out in the recliner. Throughout the hypnosis Angie appeared relaxed and calm, so I felt assured that things were going well. Little did I know that Angie was experiencing a past life.

When the session was over and I turned off the recorder and asked her to slowly open her eyes. She opened her eyes, sat up and declared, "I don't know what happened but I must have gone to sleep and had the craziest dream I have ever had! I dreamt that I was a Native American male riding for my life on horseback. I was being chased by a Native American male on horseback, but he was from a different tribe. We were at war with each other and they attacked us. We were not ready. *Oh!* He threw a hatchet and it went into the back of my head! I died. Isn't that the strangest dream you have ever heard of?"

Because of Angie's religious background, I did not tell her that she had spontaneously experienced a traumatic past life memory. It was important to me that she remained comfortable and safe. I did share with her that the hatchet landed in her head in exactly the same place that she has the migraines. Angie is now free of migraines.

Whether you believe in past lives or not, please entertain the thought that the subconscious offered a story that brought forth a healing process. Both of these women received important information, from out of the blue, about their physical bodies. The information may have come from old memories of a past existence or it might have come as a symbolic signal from the depths of the subconscious. No matter where or how the information disclosed itself, it assisted them in the healing process. Both of these stories, however, indicated the origins of their physical struggles. Both women were excited and surprised to receive this information, but they were also delighted by the positive results.

Did they carry this trauma with them from that life into this life? Maybe it wasn't a matter of carrying that burden from one life to another. It might have been a decision or choice made during their pre-life planning before they entered into this particular life. I do not know. What I do know is that it made all the sense in the world to my clients, and they were able to make physical changes because of it.

Even the most brilliant minds of our time and the most intuitive psychics cannot comprehend the magnitude of human capabilities.

Humans respond to choices in life. Do we create negatives or do we create positives? In truth, the heavens of the Universe create an epic novel that we humans are a part of.

## The Strange, the Weird, and the Wild

The following case studies are true. The people involved agreed that my perceptions were either accurate or they agreed that something profound happened. In truth, I hesitated to place this section in print. I finally decided that you must be prepared for just about anything as you venture into another person's energy field. If I perceive and experience the strange, the weird, and the wild, then you will too. Information comes to us in amazing shapes and forms. The people, even in these case studies, felt this intuitive information meant the world to them.

Jamie seemed high strung and nervous as she entered my office. She told me she felt simply terrible and needed help to get back on track. As usual, I stopped her from giving me any more information, explaining that I did not want to know anything prior to my readings. I told her that I assess a person's energy field before I am told anything verbally. She agreed.

I immediately began to move into Jamie's energy field. A dark, thick haze, like semi-transparent cellophane, surrounded her body. I pushed through it, feeling sticky as if it were clinging onto my own energy. I continued to push toward this woman's head. I felt a vibration like static electricity going in all directions and without a pattern or form. I was sensing her inability to formulate cohesive thoughts, let alone maintain them. The energy within her brain was jagged in blacks with tones of dark red.

As I scanned down into her neck I was not able to perceive any energy at all so I moved on toward her chest and heart. The entire heart chakra appeared as a cavernous hole with more inflamed black pouring out of her like a giant drain pipe. I realized I was seeing her heart gushing out a rotting substance and I could smell something metallic. I saw and smelled putrid, rotting holes in all parts of her body. The holes tunneled deep, from the outer auric field into the physical cellular body. Her liver was demolished and every other organ had a tunneling hole in it. The first chakra was completely black and I could see a great deal of negative sexual activity in her recent past. This woman was near death.

I had probably been quiet for a long period of time so I looked into her eyes and said, "How much street drugs are you doing?"

She hung her head and with a soft voice said, "I am doing a lot of cocaine. I have lost my husband and now I can no longer see my children. I am an elementary school teacher but I just lost my job there. I am living with some male friends of mine in a motel room on the west side of town."

"You are near death now. Do you realize that?" She said that she thought that might be the case but she was not willing to change anything right now. The counselor in me rose up and I did my best to assist her. We talked for a long time about her impending death, and then she slowly rose up and walked out the door.

I tried to reach her and to help her change, but I did not try to stop her from walking out the door. We must allow our clients to make their life choices and sometimes those choices happen right in front of our eyes. I remember this woman and her reading because of the dramatically ugly energy field I witnessed. While I remember every moment of this session, I do not carry any emotion about it. When you have a similar situation sitting before you, do your best, but let each person have their own path and create their own story. You cannot make changes when they are not willing to participate with you.

Eric was excited to receive a Reiki session from me. He had a delightful but intense feel about him as he eagerly jumped onto my table. I began the Reiki in my usual way, beginning at Eric's head and working downward and then back up from feet, finishing at the head where I had begun. Eric seemed quite healthy and vigorous to me.

A thought popped into my head that told me I should work more directly on his back. I began by placing one hand on his tailbone area and the other hand on the base of his skull to receive an initial overview of his spine. Immediately I saw four faces of aliens usually called the Grays! They appeared only inches from my face and seemed to be pressing toward me in a menacing way. They had the typical gray face and huge, almond-shaped black eyes that you see in the movies. This was a totally new experience for me, but I forced myself to remain still and kept my hands in place on Eric's back. I increased the Reiki energy within my own body with deliberate deep breathing and brought up the light (remember the Enrich Your Light Body exercise in Chapter Four). The faces backed away but did not leave my visual field.

I continued to build and refine my own energy field as I continued projecting it into Eric. As I changed my hand position I suddenly thought I saw something jerk from around one vertebra of his spine. I looked closer and saw that it looked like a metal clip, slightly similar to the metal clip used to hold an ace bandage wrap around an injury. Then another one and another one lifted from Eric's spine. A total of four clips lifted up from his spinal column and floated up into the air and disappeared. By the time all four clips were removed, the faces of the aliens also faded away.

I had not mentioned a word of this to Eric as it was happening. Typically, I do not speak during Reiki until I have completed the session. I then ask the person to sit in a chair as I draw a picture of their energy and what I perceived. At this point Eric had no idea what had just happened. I learned a long time ago to gently and kindly tell people what I perceive, so I hesitantly told Eric this strange story and I included the aliens.

"I knew it!" he exclaimed. "I knew that I had some type of implant or some type of control over me!" He continued excitedly, telling me about his encounters with aliens in the past.

Being a medical intuitive will require that you be ready for anything and everything. What you perceive with your clients, your friends, and relatives will sometimes have nothing to do with your own personal beliefs. Sharing your perceptions, however, whether you believe them or not, is tremendously important to the person you are assisting.

**Essential Point:**
*Sharing your perceptions, whether you believe them
or not, is tremendously important.*

My third case study happened at the very beginning of my career in energy work. In fact, as I recall, Marie was the fourth or fifth person that I ever worked with. Imagine my shock when a tiny leprechaun-like being jumped out of Marie's abdomen!

I was shy but excited to have clients in my new office space in Indianapolis. I did my best to describe Reiki to her and then asked her for permission to begin. She eagerly gave me permission so I placed my hands on her head and began the session.

When I placed my hands on her abdomen, the energy began to undulate in large waves that led to a rumbling sound. I had never experienced anything like this before. This energy seemed surprisingly different from the other areas of her body. As that thought crossed my mind, the energy field of her abdomen instantly split wide open and out jumped a two-foot-tall leprechaun-like entity. The being emitted an ear piercing screech that felt like hot needles shooting into my ears. The screeching continued as it jumped from the table onto the floor and ran hysterically around the room.

Not only was I shocked but I also had no idea what to do. Whenever I do not know what to do, I focus on the feeling of love and a vision of white light. So that is what I did. I recreated the feeling of love in my body and I visualized white light in my mind, and I blasted that energy outward in a focused laser beam toward the screaming little being. It instantly disintegrated into tiny dots of energy which then lifted up into the air and floated away.

It seemed as if the incident went on for hours but it all really happened in seconds. My hands never left Marie's abdomen during this strange occurrence. My heart thumping, I finished the Reiki session as if nothing unusual happened.

Marie sat up very slowly with an odd look on her face. "What on earth happened with my stomach! My stomach felt so weird and now I feel so different and so much better." I could not tell that woman what I saw or what I thought had taken place. I simply told her that she released a great deal of negative energy from the solar plexus and that she would probably continue to feel better in the days to come.

As a new practitioner with a new office, I did not understand what else to say or do. I could not lie to her but I did not want to terrify her either. How could I say that a screaming leprechaun gushed from her abdomen? I could only acknowledge that a release of something negative had taken place. What else could I do?

The point here is that Marie knew something important had happened. She knew a change had taken place within her, and she let me know that she recognized it. That happened in the early 1990s, and to this day I wonder if I should have described the event to this stranger or if I served her well by not informing her. Since that session I decided to tell each person about my perceptions no matter how weird or different. All has been well with that decision.

## It's Not All Disease and Drama

As you can see there are many, many influences that affect people as they live the human experience. Remember, you are entering into a person's entire story during a medical intuition reading. You may recall that these influences include our perpetual thoughts and emotions, our environment and the energetic stresses of the earth, our genetics and ancestry, past situations in our current life, as well as our past lives.

Our body and its energy field reflect the energy of relationships, people in the living world, and also people who have passed on. As a medical intuitive, this is quite a story to see, feel, sense, and merge into. How does one sort it all out? We begin by not trying to sort it all out. We simply state our perceptions and the individual will inform you what it all means.

It is a simple matter of expressing whatever you get, however you get it. It is your delivery of the information that is important. Do not slam or bombard the individual with your insights. Slow down and present your perceptions in a gentle, slow, loving manner. Use a calm, empathetic voice while expressing some of the tougher insights. Project a healing vibrational wave outward, toward the person receiving the information. It is not necessary to become serious or stern. Reflect back to your client the mood that they are feeling. In other words, if the person is laughing and having a lighthearted experience during the reading, then for goodness' sake, join in with the lightness as well. If the person is sobbing, then be there for them with sincere gentleness.

Another important guideline that I've stated before and will state again is to never interpret the information that you receive. Simply give the information as you perceive the information. Your client will tell you what it means, how it applies, and how it is affecting them. Remember the case of the woman whose head kept floating away from her body, then rolled away when it was cut off? I did not attempt to interpret that image. She told me its meaning and the effect it had on her body.

**Essential Point:**
*Do not interpret your findings, only describe them.*

Make sure that you accept your most instant impressions. The most immediate sense will be your clearest level of information because your critical, judgmental mind does not have enough time to interfere with the vibrational level of information you receive. Remember that your spirit mind is in its most unrestricted, sensitive condition when the thinking mind has not had time to move in. The logical thinking mind will negate and dissect whatever comes its way. Don't let it. Accept and trust what darts into your awareness.

Notice, right now, the sensations of your thinking mind at work as you read this book. Feel them. Recognize the sensations of them. Watch your thoughts flowing in and watch the topic of each thought. Notice now that you can switch to another channel like a radio in your vehicle. As you turn the knob, one station gives you the news that comes in consecutive logical thoughts, one after another. Turn the knob a little farther and there is only static. Turn your knob farther and you get a smooth, musical flow from a station that only plays instrumental music. Vibrations of sound flow throughout the vehicle, quietly sending you away from your thoughts and worries. You gently receive in this state of mind. You gently receive a flow. Your mind/soul feels like this.

A dear friend of mine describes it another way. He says that psychic information is like sonar in a submarine. The sub sends out a pinging wave, and that wave connects with something out in the ocean. That contact sends a different signal back to the submarine, then displays it on the sonar screen. I like that image and description too.

Connect with your spirit mind and your spirit mind will move into the cosmic soup of information like sonar. You will perceive the extraordinary, the sublime, the weird, and the unusual. You will also pick up the simple, ordinary aches and pains. You will enter into the intimate chapters of a great novel as you assist another soul on their journey.

I love to do mini readings during paranormal expos because it keeps me on my toes and I practice remaining in the constant flowing realm of the spirit mind. A young male named Mike sat down in front of me with a large grin on his face. He wanted to know if I remembered him from earlier in the year. I told him that I did remember him but had no idea what I said to him in that session. Even while he was asking me that question, I immediately saw a blazing hot line going through the right side of his jaw and I told him so. He responded, "Oh yeah . . . last night I bit down on a chicken bone and it hurt like mad." Off we went into a pertinent discussion of how he might be chewing on or ruminating on some old hurt in life.

Many people will come to you for a medical intuition reading and it will not be about disease and drama. It will be more about struggles and stresses with work, relationships, money, and the daily stuff of life. The body begins to act as an internal barometer, signaling to even the most unaware individual that something is wrong somewhere in life.

The following is an excerpt from a medical intuitive assessment. To ensure confidentiality, I will call the client Jackie.

**Tina:** If I may, I will begin with my initial comments for you and then I will ask you to comment on these first observations. The left area of your brain is absorbing information, taking in information and assimilating it in your brain. Your eyes are big and I see energy zooming into your eyes. You are really quite visual and learn visually. Your head is just lit up. I see eyes looking all over the place. It is a symbol and does not mean that everyone is looking at you. I see eyes in all kinds of different ways, and so you receive new information easily from images and the written word. This is a better way for you than listening.

It is an important symbol as well as an important sense that you use. Your head is all aglow and then around your throat and your high upper chest becomes darker like a covering over your throat and that always tells me that at least in one way, if not multiple ways, you are having a difficult time in expressing yourself. It is not just about speaking but it is also about expressing in all kinds of ways, like singing or expressing through your arms and hands because our arms are extensions of our throat area. Somehow, you expressing you is getting limited and minimized because it should be all bouncy and bright just like your head, but instead when it comes to expressing your own ideals there is some stifling. It is not rocking and rolling like all the thoughts in your mind.

I will just add one more thing too. I feel like you are already in the process of big changes because your eyes and all of these eyes around you say that you are open to new changes, but now I am feeling some anxiety inside of you. I am also sensing some level of sadness, worry, or concern that the way you are changing will affect others around you and that others will see you or know you differently. This is in your body as anxiety high up in your upper chest below your throat. You are really changing but also receiving a great deal of wisdom. You are developing into something more stately. There is a large book that you will be reading and taking in this new wisdom.

**Jackie:** Yes, I do have some anxiety. Yes, I feel it in my chest.

**Tina:** What about these eyes that I am seeing? You take in the world visually.

**Jackie:** In my college classes I never got much from the speaking parts.

**Tina:** Yes, the written word is important and reading in general is going to be very important to you.

**Jackie:** I work in a school.

**Tina:** There is an element of sadness going on with you.

**Jackie:** I have been concerned with my health and also stresses at school.

**Tina:** Would you like me to look specifically any place in your body?

**Jackie:** My head and my chest.

**Tina:** Those are the two areas I have been mentioning so far and so I will look more closely. Just allow yourself to feel open and allow me to connect in with you. Again, I am getting sadness and worry about changes around you. Instantly on the right side of your head there is a block presenting itself as a muddy red line, which is anger, and it is a pushing down and causing pressure, especially on the right side of your head.

Now the right side of our head is about bigger concepts and creativity while the left side is about details and getting things done, facts, reconciling our checkbook. There is a pushing down or against the right side of your head.

I can't imagine that you are not feeling headaches from the pushing down. It doesn't look like illness that is happening within your head. It looks like pressure from outside of you pressing down on you. It seems to be coming from life around you and it is your response to external stuff coming at you. The sinuses in your face are showing big energetic streams of tears, and when we do not cry the tears that we feel, the pressure builds up. Usually sinus problems are about holding back tears and emotions from stress and frustration and the pressure builds. There is a gushing energy pouring from your eyes and across your face. Are there tears you are not crying?

**Jackie:** Yeah, I hold a lot in.

**Tina:** Well, that takes us back to your throat area. So you see it is starting in your throat area and it's like your throat is clamping down and you are struggling and saying to yourself, "Well I can't say that or this might happen or if I really let it loose I will suffer the consequences." Now what just popped in is interesting. I am noticing that the same color of muddy, murky red from across your throat is also coming as tears from your eyes. And it's that color of anger. Even if you tell me there is not an angry bone in your body, I would have to say that you are full of anger but especially frustration pushing down on the right side of your head and plugged up in your face and the same dark red is gushing out of your eyes and across your face. Why are you holding in so much?

**Jackie:** It is because of my work and I am trying to keep it in and not to cause problems.

**Tina:** You have brought up work multiple times now so ask me a specific question about work and I will see what I get.

**Jackie:** Will I be working in the school next year?

**Tina:** I feel like you are but the question pops up, do you really want to be?

**Jackie:** Well, I work two jobs so I have to hold onto both until I see.

**Tina:** But the school in particular—I do not feel any movement so I do not feel any movement for you away from school but the question keeps popping up in my mind—do you really want to remain there in this school? Because as I look at you and then the school it looks heavy and dense to me. You are bright and as I look toward you, you look really good but this school looks heavy and dense and it appears as the same muddy color as inside of your head. What pops up about this for you?

**Jackie:** Mostly it is just stress. It is the people that are causing the stress.

**Tina:** Do you want to ask about the other job?

**Jackie:** Yes.

**Tina:** Gosh, your other job looks so much brighter. It is almost as bright as you are. It is really up there. Good grief. Now I am seeing a pale rainbow bridge between you and the other job. Does it feel this positive to you?

**Jackie:** Only when two certain people are not there!

**Tina:** Give me their first names only.

**Jackie:** Bob and Randy.

**Tina:** Here is what I get: their goals are to climb the ladder. A ladder appeared and they are climbing the ladder and at the same time they are stepping on the heads of others to climb it. Does that fit what is happening?

**Jackie:** Yep! (She giggles.)

**Tina:** Isn't this all amazing?

**Jackie:** Yes, it is.

**Tina:** They are very self-focused and their own light is not very bright. There is a film around them. They are down inside of themselves and cannot see anyone else. Now Jackie, if you could just let them be who they are and let them be buttheads about things. The higher ups at work are seeing your light and they already know that the buttheads are being buttheads. I don't know why I am calling them buttheads, but it feels right to call them this. Your light is so bright that you are not getting overlooked. You are not invisible to them. Does this make sense to you? How are they getting to you?

**Jackie:** They just want power and I just want to do my job and have a good time and all they care about is the power. Yes, they are buttheads.

**Tina:** Now, you are clamping down your words in your throat in this job too.

**Jackie:** No, you are correct. I don't there either.

**Tina:** Jackie, the energy is so low in your throat that if this keeps up you will find yourself with an illness and it will begin to affect you physically. People begin to get a lot of sore throats and thyroid problems and that kind of thing. I do not see that you are having physical problems right now, but when I look deeper into your throat I see hands clamping down on you. Someone really wants you to keep your mouth shut. You might feel you are in jeopardy but you are not in jeopardy.

Your work at school looks much darker than your second job. You cannot stop the crumbling. If you need to, go more with the flow of the changes and not buck the system. Go with the flow. The more you worry about your jobs, the more your body thinks it really happened. I have to tell you that you must catch yourself in the worry thoughts and make yourself change it. This is always going to work out. Every time a door closes, I know that three or five or ten doors will open, but you will not notice them if you do not get in control of your worry thoughts. You are angry but even more importantly there is sadness and worry, worry, worry. If I focus on the closed doors, I cannot even see the open ones. This is making sense to you, isn't it?

**Jackie:** Yes, it makes all kinds of sense.

**Tina:** I can really hear the lightness in your voice. I can hear you perking up.

**Jackie:** Mostly I've been worried about the pressure in my head and chest, but now I am not so worried.

**Tina:** I want you to focus on getting into control because right now you don't think you have any control or any choice. Things are crumbling with the two buttheads. I love calling them buttheads. You need to shift the focus on you and cry when you feel it and express by writing a letter that you promise not to mail. Write it to express yourself without any censoring. Promising yourself not to mail it will give you permission to say everything.

Now let me look at your heart. I see this darkness that is pushing down on the organ of your heart because of stuffing things. There is a box around your heart and then pressure against the box. It is smashing down on your heart. Your heart is fluttering and missing beats.

**Jackie:** Yes, you are right.

**Tina:** Our bodies do not know fear. Emotions come from thoughts. When there are more negatives in our thoughts, it ends up in our body. Make yourself change your mind and feel the relief. You think you are boxed in.

**Jackie:** Yeah, I feel trapped in with my work.

**Tina:** I want you to go into work tonight as a fascinated observer and watch the people around you. The clear observer is fascinated but neutral. They do not react with emotion. Their detachment allows for clarity. Can you go into work tonight and do that?

**Jackie:** Yes, I will.

You can see that this session was not about disease, potential death, or even aliens. Many of your readings will be centered around everyday situations like Jackie's. Remember that sometimes there is no disease or pathology to find. Not all of them will be remarkable or weird. While many of the people that you assist will feel divine intervention just happened, you will think that the session was quite ordinary. Notice that Jackie was not ill at all, at least not at this point. She was experiencing a great deal of stress and was aware of an irregular heart beat and headaches. She was relieved to have some guidance about its source and how to possibly handle the struggles.

Illness will present itself in the energy field first and as it becomes more solid, building up more substance, it will begin to appear in the physical body. I spent some of Jackie's session assisting her to make some tiny achievable steps to alleviate her stress, but it is up to her to make different choices and changes in her life. You can only offer guidance. If she chooses not to make even tiny changes, you as the practitioner must allow that. If you begin to carry any responsibility for your clients, you will begin to deteriorate with them. If you find yourself working hard to get your clients to make healthy changes, you are actually carrying more and more of their burdens, and they are not yours to carry.

Esther Hicks succinctly described it this way in a workshop in San Diego, California, on February 15, 2003: "You cannot get sick enough to help people get better. You cannot get poor enough to help people thrive. It is only in your thriving that you have anything to offer anyone. If you're wanting to be of an advantage to others, be as tapped in, tuned in, and turned on as you can possibly be."

Carrying the burdens of others will deplete you. Let each have their own choices and make their own decisions. You simply cannot make another person change. The more you try, the more you will deteriorate. Allow each person—yes, even a loved one—to have their own path and their own way of taking that path. You can share your knowledge with people, even your loved ones, but you cannot make them follow through. No matter how well meaning and knowledgeable you are, if you push and push you will only receive resentment back. Each person insists on living their own way at their own pace.

### Essential Point:
*Carrying the burdens of others will deplete you.*

You see, it is not all disease and drama. If you find yourself searching only for illnesses and looking only for despair, you will also be missing a great deal of the entire story. Look for the individual's development, the person's strengths, gifts, and assets. Each person before you, no matter how ill or stressed they are, also carries wisdom.

Enter into a relationship with their wisdom. Along with the tough information, share the positive information you perceive and emphasize those qualities. Each person needs to hear there is hope in rough times. Don't allow them to leave you in despair. Even as you describe very intimate struggles or severe illness, it is up to you to present it in a healing manner and to give each person faith and the expectation that they will succeed toward well-being.

# PART THREE

Medical Intuition in Action

# Chapter Ten

## Rising into Action

So far, this entire training course has established a foundation to become a precise medical intuitive. You have been accumulating a great deal of information and activating all of your intuitive senses. If you have participated with the steps along the way, you have participated in a profound and intimate development within yourself. This development will sustain you through many personal situations and many experiences with the world around you. Do you remember and understand the depth of this process and especially the progress you have created?

Here is the next step in your process.

Go back and review your entire journal. You will read and see the changes that you have already made. As you review your journal, take time to notice everything that has happened before you move forward, absorbing and assimilating your evolution thus far.

### Your X-ray Abilities: Taking Action

We have the ability to direct our energy field outward and the energetic body responds to our powerful focused thought. We have discussed and practiced the creation of clear mental intent earlier in this book, and the projection of your elastic energy body into a laser beam of energy. Your laser beam has hypersensitive sensors at its outer edge. Medical intuitives set their intent to project the elastic energy body outward like warm stretched taffy toward the client's energy and to their physical body.

**Essential Point:**
*Medical intuitives set intent, then project the elastic*
*energy body outward like warm stretched taffy.*

Remember the experience earlier in this book when you practiced getting in charge of your energy? You sent your energy outward and upward to deliberately sit on the roof. Remember how I asked you to control yourself and not fly around haphazardly? Remember how you practiced until you could move your energy in a deliberate, precise way? It is time now to utilize that ability and project your energy for the purpose of medical intuition.

X-ray vision requires that you project your energy field outward and into the physical body of the receiver/client. To do this effectively, we must learn to control the projection, control how we project, when we project, and where we project. It is not so much the concentration of thought but the concentration of energy. The laser-like form of your energy field beams outward, surveys the aura, penetrates the skin, and probes deeper into the body tissue to receive an image, a feeling, or a perception regarding the individual. The laser beam of focused energy resembles the power of an x-ray machine visualizing and offering a more complete internal assessment. Return to Chapter Five to review the steps for creating your laser beam.

**Essential Point:**
*Medical intuitives set the intent with a laser-like*
*concentration of energy, not the*
*concentration of thoughts.*

Let's begin to know our x-ray machine capabilities by engaging in some play. Remember that intuition will always present itself as childlike imagination. The more you play, the more precise your abilities will be. The more playful and relaxed you are, the greater your abilities are to access vibrationally based information. When you accept and trust the most instant impressions that pop in, you are accepting the clearest information.

Here is a simple drawing of the bones inside of a human arm and hand. Study this picture until you feel as if you have memorized it for this experience. Do not move onto the practice steps until you are confident that you can see the image of the bones in your inner mind. When you have memorized it, close your eyes and imagine the bone structures in your mind's eye.

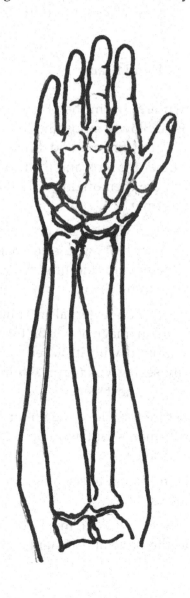

Prepare to document in your journal anything that rushes into your awareness. Read through all of the following steps before doing this practice exercise. Then go back and read each step individually and put it into practice. Stop and document each step along the way. Your documentation might be colors, feelings, words, images, movement, energy, or knowing. It is important to understand that there is no way to do this incorrectly. Simply notice.

## Steps for the Arm and Hand Scan

1. Place your own arm, from the elbow to your hand, on a table before you. Slowly study the look of your arm—its shape, the skin, the fingers and fingernails. Study your arm and remember the look and the feel of it stretched out before you. You are memorizing only the external look of your arm at this time.

2. Remember how you studied the object in the room earlier in this course? Apply that process now. Close your eyes and imagine the skin, fingers, and fingernails and the shape of your arm in your mind's eye.

3. Repeat the study of your external arm until your mind's eye quickly produces an image of it. Don't work at this practice exercise. Play around with it. When you realize that you are successfully seeing your arm within your mind's eye then move on to the next step.

4. Study the picture provided again of the typical bone structure of a human's arm and hand. Allow it to imprint in your mind as before.

5. Create a powerful intent to see like an x-ray machine then relax any effort about it.

6. Now push your energy field, in a laser-like beam, past the skin, down to the bone and imagine seeing like an x-ray machine.

7. Repeat these steps again and again until you know that you are witnessing your bones within your arm and hand. Document your impressions.

8. Notice the sensations of seeing internally. Play without any effort as you imagine the bone structure.

9. Now look again and send a laser beam of focused energy into the joints of the elbow, then the wrist and then the fingers. Simply notice, without judgment, whatever comes up.

10. After sensing something about the different joints, document your awareness.

11. Now envision the muscles and tissue all around the bones. What is your sense of the muscles and how do they instantly appear to you?

12. Now repeat the process for your other arm. Are they equal or is there a difference?

Describe and draw your perceptions in your journal now.

The next step is to playfully practice on someone's arm other than your own. Take the pressure off of yourself. Inform the people that you are a student and need to practice. If you do not feel you have anyone you can ask directly then remember to ask someone telepathically. Ask for permission to look deeply into one of their arms (not the entire body yet). When you receive permission, playfully imagine that you are seeing the bones and tissue of their forearm. Then repeat the practice by looking into the other arm of that person. Do the arms appear equal or are they different? Document any awareness, no matter how miniscule, that pops into your mind. Then go to another person and ask for permission, and another and another, each time practicing the projection of your energy field and recording your awareness in detail.

Important: At this point, focus only on arms and hands until you feel and know you are successfully projecting your energy outward and inward. The focus of this experience is to learn to project your intent and deliberately control your energy field.

## Progressing to the Next Level

Progressing to the next stage of medical intuition is a fascinating time of discovery. Here we will go beyond visualizing bones and joints and venture into a more meaningful phase of intuition. Hopefully you have practiced your x-ray skills on your own arm and hand and then practiced with the arms of other people. As you increase your abilities to notice subtle, tiny details, you might have noticed that each arm presented a different feel or image or sensation. No two people are alike and no two energy fields are alike. Review the subtle differences that you have already picked up with different people.

While each person as a whole vibrates in unique ways, so too does each illness within each individual. Examples of illness, such as high blood pressure or an earache, have their own vibrational patterns. However, because each illness also resides within the unique energy field of an individual, it will have another layer of unique characteristics. X-ray vision will convey those differences to you if you remain alert to it.

## The Next Step

Make a list of people you know who have a diagnosed illness. Ask those people for permission to scan their bodies to see what their particular diagnosis looks like to you. Remember that you can verbally or psychically ask each one for their permission. When you receive a firm, undeniable yes to your request, you can write each person's name with diagnosis on a separate page in your journal. Begin with people who have already been diagnosed with a certain illness or disorder. It does not matter what type of illness it is. For example, it could be a sinus infection, asthma, cancer, strep throat, a broken toe, etc.

The illness does not need to be dramatic or life threatening.

For now, practice only with people who have received an official diagnosis by a physician. Ask each person where the illness is located unless the illness affects an entire system. In that case, ask the individual what system is affected by that illness.

Constantly practice with every person that you know or hear about. Make sure that you know the diagnosis and what part of the body is affected. This will make a great deal of sense when you think about it. Practicing with people who have a predetermined diagnosis will help you learn about the energy signature of that particular illness and how that information consistently comes to you. You will also begin to naturally pick up other intuitive information about each person as you scan for a particular diagnosis.

**Essential Point:**
*Asking permission will ensure you are*
*working with integrity.*

Consider for a moment all the people you know who have some condition that has been medically diagnosed. Who do you know at work that talks about having high blood pressure or diabetes? Which of your friends or family always complain of exhaustion or are in constant pain? Who do you know that has been diagnosed with depression? Find all the people you can who have been diagnosed with heart problems. Do you have a nephew with a broken leg or a neighbor with gout? Who do you know that is recently recovering from surgery of any type? There is no end to the maladies around you.

It is imperative that you actually take the time to work with a multitude of people to specifically assess pre-determined diseases or disorders. This step is crucial in accelerating your skills and solidifying your x-ray abilities.

Finding two or more people with the same diagnosis will enhance your skills even more. Two people with the same diagnosis will offer you an opportunity to distinguish the subtle differences I mentioned earlier. Again, each person, as a whole, vibrates in unique ways; thus, so too does each illness within each individual vibrate uniquely. Utilize this opportunity to distinguish subtle differences in visual images and insights from one person to another.

### Essential Point:
*Each person, as a whole, vibrates in unique ways; thus, so too does each illness within each individual vibrate uniquely.*

## How to Begin and End Sessions

For years I have noticed that professional psychics and mediums are frequently ill or even hospitalized. At psychic fairs I have noticed that most of the intuitives who are lined up to do mini readings, are haggard looking. Their skin as well as their aura is gray with very little vitality emanating from their body or mind. Something is not right with this picture.

After many conversations with other intuitives, I came to an understanding that is somewhat mind-blowing. Intuitives must be extremely careful in how we begin and end each and every session. We are sloppy with our words and our energetic cleanliness.

First of all, we must be exact in who or what we call out for. In other words, if you simply ask the Universe for help, you may not necessarily receive the best help available. If we did not deliberately and thoughtfully request the specific and precise assistance we want, then we may receive just any spirit person floating by at the time. It sounds funny when I say that, but it is a critical component in one's intuitive work.

Each word, each phrase, and each sentence we declare is of vital importance. What we think, say aloud, or intuitively request will return back to us exactly with the same frequency that we sent out. As intuitives, we create and then send out a unique, intense energetic connection with each person we work with. This connection is real and powerful and is tapped into each client. Intuitives begin sessions with a type of energetic cording to connect into the person's eternal story. We then bring the session to a close and move on to our next appointment.

No one, and I mean no one, ever pulls their energy back from the client at the end of each session. We intuitives are leaving energetic threads or cords with each person that we work with. These threads allow some level of energy exchange back and forth between you and every human for the remainder of everyone's lives and possibly even after this life.

As a result, the intuitive is not living clean and clear within their own energy field. Our body, mind, spirit, and soul remain dramatically influenced by the many, many people we have worked with. How can we maintain our own health when we are under the constant barrage of thoughts, emotions, and traumatic events from other people's lives? They are also affected by our life and every other intuitive they have worked with as well.

During a session with me, a well-known professional psychic who was struggling with cancer made the following comment:

"I *love* the part where you point out the difference between the temporary energetic psychic connections we use in our work and the more permanent connections that build up over time in our general relationships! I had never considered that before, but it certainly seems right, and I can feel the difference within myself."

We need to disconnect from our clients to avoid this dilemma. We need to create good clean closure at the end of each session and at the end of our work day. We also must also release the threads from every person we have ever worked with in the past. The new steps listed below are the most important pieces of information in this entire book. By taking these steps, you will be caring for yourself in the most profound way. You will also be saving your own life. And I mean that.

**Steps for a Medical Intuitive Session**

Here are point-by-point steps for a medical intuitive session. Feel free to copy it to have on hand as you perform a medical intuitive assessment.

**Point-by-Point Steps for a Medical Intuitive Session**

1.  Have colored markers and the human drawing or the assessment form ready. Have a digital recorder and computer on hand if you are comfortable recording your session.

2.  **(New information!)** At the beginning of each session, ask that a sacred space be placed around you and your client for the most perfect work and healing to happen. Do not create the space yourself. Ask that your specialty guide create the perfect sacred and safe space for the work that is about to happen. You may feel it or you may be able to see it. Intuitively invite each client to join you in that sacred space.

3.  Do not try hard to do anything. Only passively notice whatever comes in. It will always feel like imagination, like you are merely making it up.

4.  Do an instant self-assessment to evaluate your own body, mind, and emotions.

5.  Begin to shift your awareness. You are soul energy with a spirit mind, more than a brain with a physical body. Your eyes can be open or closed—whatever is comfortable for you.

6.  Call in your specialty guide to assist you specifically with medical intuition. Merge your efforts together.

7.  Sit, notice your thoughts, and then quiet your mind.

8.  Stop thinking of yourself. Become the neutral observer.

9.  Release all thoughts about you and direct all awareness to the other person.

10. Ask each person for permission to proceed.

11. Expand your energy beyond your skin. Feel the non-physical you.

12. Lock onto the intent for powerful x-ray vision.

13. Feel and see your energy forming into the shape of a laser beam.

14. Allow your energy to project outward in front of you.

*Face-to-face session:* Project your energy to the receiver and envelop them.

*Phone session:* Project your energy outward toward their name and their voice. It will feel like you are following along an energy wave from their voice and name. Repeat their name over and over in your mind as you project it outward.

15. Move your energy beam around the outer aura of the person.

16. Trust and accept your most immediate impressions. You are picking up the story of this person.

17. Report all information to the person.

18. Notice instant sensations and physical feelings within your own body. These are really signals about the individual you are working with.

19. Notice any instant thoughts that pop into your mind. It is information about them, not you.

20. Notice instant images or colors that come to you even if they seem shadowy and elusive. Look at the energy field from head to toe. You might see it as a generalized human form.

21. Notice the actions of any images you see. The action or non-action gives you more information about this person and their life.

22. When you feel you have assessed the outer aura you can move on.

23. If you are strongly drawn to a certain location within the body, go with that pull no matter where it takes you. If you are not drawn to a certain place, then begin to send your laser beam scan deep into the head and brain, eyes, sinuses, ears, and jaw.

24. Divide the body into sections. Look into the chakras, the organs, and surrounding tissue.

25. Go deep within the neck, throat, and shoulders and down the arms and into the hands.

26. Bring awareness back to the chest, looking into the lungs first before the heart. (The heart energy is very prominent, so look into the lungs first so you do not miss this area.)

27. Now scan the organ and chakra of the heart.

28. Continue throughout the abdomen, scanning each chakra and each organ.

29. Scan throughout the hip and groin area.

30. Go into each leg, each joint, all the way to the toes.

31. Scan the bones and the spine.

32. Look at body systems in general such as blood, muscles, lymph, etc.

33. Ask the person if there is any place in their body that they would like you to view more specifically.

34. Bring your session to a close, always emphasizing the positive aspects and also wisdom presented by your guide or the individual's guide.

35. **(New information!)** At the close of each session, or at least at the end of each day, invite a specialty guide who excels in cleaning and clearing to create the ideal cleansing filter through which you can return to maintain perfect health for you. Deliberately and consciously pull your energetic laser beam back from the client and the experience through the filter. You may feel the filter or you may actually

see it working. You can assist yourself by inhaling and imagining that each inhalation pulls your energy back to you through that filter. A possible command to use at the same time might be, "I now bring me and only me back to me, clean and clear, through a perfect filter provided for me by my divine cleansing specialist". Sometimes I see a thick substance clinging to the filter. I am so comforted and pleased to know that I am not bringing someone else's emotional density into my life.

This is my newest information and the biggest tip of all! I am learning and evolving constantly and so are you. When I originally published *Become a Medical Intuitive* in 2012, I had not received the new steps presented above, so I am now delighted to present more detailed information in this revision.

## An Overall Prospective of Medical Intuitive Sessions

Can you see that there is no end to the opportunities to practice seeing with x-ray eyes? Do not fool yourself into thinking that you do not have anyone to practice with. That is only old fear raising its ugly head, trying to stop your success and keep you in your old, known place. There truly is no end point to our medical intuitive education.

When you begin this portion of your development you will be bombarded with opportunities. You will not be able to keep it all straight unless you document each situation. Log in each with as much detail as you can to give you a truer sense of your advancing skill level. Carry your journal with you so you are always prepared, because the opportunities are everywhere.

You will also discover that focusing on pre-diagnosed conditions actually opens the door to all levels of medically based intuition. Centering on a diagnosis that is already determined builds confidence and gives you a foundation of knowledge. That foundation will create a bridge for you to transition naturally and expand into the whole experience of human health and well-being.

That bridge will take you from a novice to a medical intuitive professional.

You have practiced all of the experiences throughout this book and have taken the steps to document all of your awareness along the way. Taking the time to put this awareness into action refines your intent to excel at medical intuition. The old adage "Practice makes perfect" applies in medical intuition. Skill and accuracy develops when you work with medical intuition for a multitude of people on a daily basis. Practice, practice, and practice some more. The repetition will enhance your skillful awareness of the energetic body. Take the time to build and excel as a skilled medical intuitive.

**Essential Point:**
*Project your intent and deliberately control*
*your energy field.*

Review your journal again to reinforce all that you have achieved. This book has offered you a progressive, step-by-step program to discover and to enrich your natural medical intuitive talents. It is time now to begin using those talents. It is important to realize that x-ray vision is not the only skill used within a medical intuitive reading. The session entails many aspects of a professional occasion. Let's walk through the general process of medical intuition together now. After this general process, we will look at each step along the way to deepen your understanding and enhance your own abilities. The following steps are the same for distance work, phone sessions, or readings in your office. Let's start at the beginning of a medical intuition session.

You are about to do a medical intuitive reading. Any second now. the person you are expecting will walk in for an office visit or the phone will ring and you will pick it up for a distant reading. How and where will you begin?

Prepare your room so it nourishes and enhances your spirit mind. Are the lights correct? Is there a healing ambiance for you and your visitors? Have magic markers and a pen ready to draw and write down your perceptions. You can use the blank human form or the medical intuition scanning form, both of which are provided for you in this book. You may also want to digitally record your findings in conjunction with a drawing, so have a digital recorder and a computer ready to download and burn a CD for the individual. When you progress as a medical intuitive, you will be flooded with information in the first minutes of each session, so be prepared.

Before the individual walks into your room or calls you on the phone, you must first assess your own body, mind, and emotions. How are you feeling at this moment? Are you happy, a little depressed, tired, or energized? Do you have aches or pains anywhere in your own body? This initial assessment of your own body status should become the standard. Do not make a big deal of it. This needs to be a fast review of where you are emotionally and what is happening physically within your own body.

Your self-evaluation can be an instant assessment. Just check in and know yourself first before you merge your energy with another person. For example, if you do not notice that you are having sinus pressure in the left side of your head prior to the session, you might later misidentify that symptom as a signal from your client's energy field. Making this quick self-scan immediately provides you a level of clarity before moving into a reading for your client.

Your personal assessment also provides you with a more profound sense that you really are more soul energy than a physical body. You have already prepared by practicing the steps for creating a daydreamlike mind and the steps for creating powerful intent. You are a soul with a spirit mind more than you are a brain with a physical body. You begin to merge into the neutral observer of the spirit mind. Call in your specialty guide specifically for each and every client, asking for assistance in providing the clearest information and the highest good for the person you are about to assist.

**Essential Point:**
*You are soul energy with a spirit mind more
than a brain with a physical body.*

Each step in the medical intuitive process is the same, whether
you sit down with an individual in person or on the phone. Greet
them pleasantly to help put them at ease. Remember, they might
be nervous or afraid. Ask for permission to begin the session. Wait
for an answer. Even when the person has come to me voluntarily
and is physically sitting before me, I still ask permission. This, in
fact, encourages the person receiving the assessment to actively
participate with the process that is about to happen. I inform them
that they do not lose control and they can actually block me out
if they choose, and I will not be able to pick up any information
for them. I ask them to feel very open and fascinated about
the adventure we are going on together. Can you see how that
comment places them in an active role?

Now notice your thoughts zooming all over the place and
just let them zoom. While your thoughts are rushing around,
focus on the true purpose of what you want to accomplish in this
particular moment. Notice that your mind wants to stay in charge
so your thoughts might scurry around even more now. Notice
without judgment. Judgment sends your thoughts flinging into
wildness. The mind loves judgment because it regains control. If
you are critical of your client or yourself, your left brain remains
in control. If you move into fear or worry, your left brain is still in
control. Any thoughts about yourself should be a signal that you
are not in your spirit mind. This time is all about the person who
wants your help. You begin by concentrating on your energy but
not necessarily your thoughts. Can you feel the difference?

Turn each reading over to your spirit guide and your spirit
mind. Notice a sensation of settling into your dreamy spirit mind,
allowing your spirit guide's information to come forth. Clearly
ask your guide for accurate and distinct clarity as you begin your
assessment. Relax and feel yourself becoming passive but keenly
aware. In other words, you are not putting forth any effort to do

anything or accomplish anything. Give it to Spirit. Do not push or try hard to do this. It is all about noticing and not toiling, sensing and not taking action. Feel the difference?

Remember the experience of sending your energy up through the ceiling and sitting on the roof? Medical intuition offers the same experience and that same playfulness. Do not take yourself so seriously. Feel and imagine a laser beam of focused energy building inside of you. Feel your intent as a medical intuitive building within you. Allow your awareness to move into a high sensitivity. The medical intuitive then locks onto the feeling of x-ray vision.

Feel or see your energy forming into the shape of a laser beam. Create the feeling of a laser beam rather than the thought of it. Project your energy by pushing it outward in front of you, toward the person you are working with. Feel and imagine that beam rocketing out of your entire body toward the individual. If this is a phone session, send the laser beam outward toward the sound of their voice and the vibration of their name. Names and voices carry a person's energetic signature. Repeat their name over and over in your mind to solidify that connection.

### Essential Point:
*Creating the feeling as well as the thought of a laser beam heightens its strength and ability to receive.*

You will instantly pick up insights and information. All of these factors will rush into your awareness in the first minute of connection. Go with the most instant information. Trust it no matter how odd it is or how mundane it might seem. Move your vision around the aura, sensing or viewing within your mind's eye from the back of your eyelids or from the center of your head.

Discuss each insight or each psychic signal with the person that sits before you. Feel the flow. Look around, taking note, drawing it, and describing whatever pops into your mind. Feel the effortlessness on your part, as if you are a docile, neutral bystander taking in the environment. Take note of everything that you instantly detect. Take note of your most immediate, instinctual awareness as you enter into their personal story. The following questions offer you guidelines to look for in the first minutes of a reading:

- How do I suddenly feel emotionally?
- What changes do I instantly feel in my own body? (These are only energy signatures of your client and not your own issues.)
- What do I suddenly know that seems to come out of nowhere?
- Are there distant sounds around the person?
- What colors appear?
- What vibrational information is in the colors?
- Do I suddenly smell something that was not there before?
- What actions or movement or lack of action is there?
- What do I rapidly notice about the energy form?
- What am I noticing about the general vitality and size of the person's energy form, the aura? What colors are present, and are they dull or bright? Where are they located?
- Are there any places on this person that seem devoid of energy or color?
- Is there any sense of other people involved with this person, either negatively or positively? Are there any other human forms nearby? How does the human(s) appear?
- What action or non-action do you notice?

Look all around the auric field. There is no end to the initial intuitive information that floats within it. The initial information may seem to be located within the auric field because you have not yet entered into the physical body. When the most immediate flooding of information seems to wane, you will know it is time to shift your awareness deeper into their physical body. Again, lock onto the idea that your intent is a powerful x-ray vision for your client. Feel or see your energy forming into the shape of a laser beam. Notice the feel of the beam rather than the thought of it.

Now create your laser beam sensor and continue to move through the aura, entering into the individual's physical body. Feel or see your sensors pushing past the skin, then down inside of the person. If you are strongly drawn to a certain location within the body, go with that pull no matter where it takes you. If you are not drawn immediately to a certain area, then begin at the head.

Divide the person's body into sections for viewing. Begin with the head and work downward throughout the body, all the way to the toes and the soles of the feet. Look into each chakra, each organ and surrounding tissue. I recommend that when you enter the chest area, you specifically look into the lungs before the heart. The heart chakra and the actual organ of the heart usually hold a great deal of information. Remember that the HeartMath Institute states that the heart muscle is made up of the same cells that are found in the brain. Because of this, the heart tends to hold dramatic information. The strength of this information may cause you to focus on the heart and forget about the lungs. If you create a pattern of assessing the lungs prior to the heart, you will be less likely to overlook the remainder of the chest.

### Essential Point:
*View the lungs before the heart.*

While your laser beam focus instantly picks up x-ray images, your five physical senses are receiving information as well. You will spontaneously see, smell, hear, touch, and know a great deal of information. Accept the waves of knowing because they are truly your natural sixth sense. Notice natural connections between all aspects and details that jump into your mind.

As you bring the session to a close, ask if there is a physical location the client would like you to scan even more deeply. Make sure that the person does not tell you why to look more closely. Refocus your laser beam and go into that area with even more precision, looking for even more detail. Discuss your more detailed findings first, then explore their reasons for asking you to do this. Bring the session to a close, always emphasizing to the client the positive aspects that were discovered and any teachings presented by spirit guides. Also *always* remember to bring your own energy back through the filter provided to you by your guide to assure you make a clean and neutral release of this person.

**Essential Point:**
*As you bring the session to a close, ask if there is any physical location they would like you to scan even more deeply.*

Take your most immediate impressions as the most accurate because the thinking mind does not have time to interfere with judgment or criticism. Do not work hard at this. Can you *feel* that toiling and straining is profoundly different than observing, noticing, and perceiving? The difference is enormous and enormously important. Passively detecting as a calm spectator is vital to success as a medical intuitive. Feel the neutral observer within you. Yes, there is a sensation of neutrality. The neutral observer has nothing to gain personally and has no emotion, so the neutral observer sees and understands from a clearer perspective. Again, do not work, strain, or toil over these steps and the goal. It is all about noticing and bringing back each thought that has strayed, then doing it again with fascination, not labor.

Remember that doing medical intuition work with a person sitting in front of you is no different than doing the assessment for a person on the other side of the world. Energy is not affected by distance. Utilize the same steps for medical intuition for a distance of inches or thousands of miles.

**Essential Point:**
*Utilize the same steps for a distance of inches or
thousands of miles.*

## An Intimate Session with Doris

I had Doris on the phone to schedule an appointment. She specifically requested that the reading focus on her physical body and the struggles that she had been having. I stopped her right there and asked her to refrain from telling me anything prior to the reading. She was stunned and said it was difficult for her to remain quiet when her struggles were so consuming. I told her I could understand her discomfort, but it was important that I not hear her diagnosis or her symptoms ahead of time. I informed her that it would interfere with my psychic clarity. Doris began to giggle, so I knew she liked the idea.

I, myself, do not want any information ahead of time because it seems to only get in my way psychically. The more I know about the client, the less accurate and informative I am. I do not want any facts, details, ideas, or history about the client, and I also do not want to hear it from a concerned friend. For instance, a client may begin to tell me about a friend who they think will be interested in making an appointment with me. I interrupt and insist that they not tell me anything about their friend ahead of time and suggest they simply tell their friend what I do and let the friend make an appointment if it feels right to them.

It delights me to see people's reactions when I refuse to take advantage of the information being offered. I rely on my impressions and I trust the ones that fly into my head as if out of nowhere. I insist on expecting Spirit to be there for me and the individual I am working with, and I insist on trusting the information that comes. I also do not want the client to think I did an Internet search about them or that I made up the entire reading based on the information they told me about themselves.

When I schedule an appointment I do not ask for their last name or their address. I only ask them to account for the different time zones and inform them that I am on Eastern Time in the United States so they can adjust the appointment time to wherever they are. I do ask for a phone number just in case of an emergency and the need to reschedule.

About one week later Doris called me at the scheduled time. I asked her to simply sit quietly with me and feel very open and even excited about the reading. We sat together quietly for probably less than a minute. I began extending my energy toward the feel of Doris and to the sound of her voice when we greeted each other. To me, it feels as if I am walking into the same room that this person is sitting in and saying hi and introducing myself to them. I am actually projecting my sense of self or my energy outward to that person.

The following is what happened, how I processed my perceptions, what I said to Doris, and how she confirmed my findings.

I began to see a very vague outline of a human form, the head, shoulders, and torso. My attention was drawn to her chest area where there was a heavy red maroon color in the shape of a square. The shape actually reminded me of a heavy shield across the front of her body. As I have mentioned before, muddy or thick burgundy or maroon color is how the vibration of anger and pain appear to me. I told Doris that she may not be aware of anger, but she had a shield of anger across her chest and heart area.

### Essential Point:
*The detailed characteristics of color*
*will give you detailed information.*

As I said this to her, I immediately saw a very large white daisy opening wide, then partially closing and opening once again. I always tell my clients the images I get and what information I get from those images. The daisy showed that Doris had been working on her issues beneath the protective shield. The fact that the flower actually took an action is even more revealing. The opening and closing movement told me that her heart was beginning to open up to the world but closed back up when she hesitated and became afraid. I told Doris that the opening and closing of the daisy seemed to be moving with the rhythm of her breathing. I said that she was literally taking in the breath of life into her body, but the thickened shield was getting in the way for that to consistently happen.

The action or non-action of a symbol gives vital information about the person. For example, the daisy could have opened and then shriveled up and blown away. What would you have made of that action if you had visualized that? What a different symbol and what a different message that would have been for her!

**Essential Point:**
*The action or non-action of a symbol*
*gives vital information.*

As I peered into her energy field, her form kept slipping over to the right of my screen of vision. Instead of thinking something was wrong with me, I instead told Doris that I believed she was uncomfortable with the direct attention that she was receiving during this reading and that it might be hard for her. I described how her energetic form stood before me one moment but quickly slid to the side. She slowly came back into my vision only to slide away again. She giggled and agreed that this much direct attention was very difficult for her. She said she would try to be more comfortable for the remainder of the session because it was so interesting to her already. I told Doris that a reading is a very special, intimate time for someone, and I asked that she allow it to happen. Guess what? She stopped slipping away and we continued on with the session.

I noticed that the energy around her neck and throat was dark and quite diminished. I described this image to her and told Doris that the throat is about expressing our individual truth through our words, our arms and hands, through singing or writing, etc.

"This area around your neck is very congested and is somewhat blocked." As I said those words aloud, the energy from Doris's head and neck shifted from a vague, washed-out shade of violet to a bright rich, deep purple shining out in all directions. I described this immediate change to her and how the reading was already assisting her. I informed her that I could see that she was actively listening and processing the information.

As the aura around and throughout her head continued to glow, I was instantly drawn to her legs, which were completely void of color. There was no energy flowing in them at all! Then her arms and legs became pine cones. I shared with Doris that her skin was rough, dry, and scaly like a pine cone. I also told her that I had been scratching my own skin throughout the reading and did not realize it until now. My own body had begun itching as I picked up energetic signals from this client. Picking up intuitive information in this manner is common and does not mean that you are taking on their energy or their problems. You are receiving only the information and not the other person's malady.

I was then drawn to Doris's groin area and the base of her spine. Dark, blackish energy was shooting out of her first chakra. I continued to watch dark energy shooting from her hip and groin area one minute, then the next minute rushing back toward the groin area then bouncing away. Even though my mind kept hearing the word "vagina," I kept using the word "groin" as I described all of this to Doris. Then Spirit began to yell "vagina" inside of my head and it would not stop until I finally said, "Doris, I keep calling this everything but what I need to call it. I need to tell you that this is all about your vagina and your sensuality and your sexuality!"

And Doris, bless her heart, responded, "Well, you need to tell it like it is!" These were words of wisdom from Doris.

I finally listened to the guidance from Doris and Spirit and said these words out loud: "Doris, you have been blocking out your femininity and your sexuality. You are a sensual being and you have not been paying attention to this aspect of yourself, and in fact you have been blocking it out. There, I said it."

**Essential Point:**
*Use a gentle, sensitive voice as you share
sensitive information.*

I glanced at the clock for the first time and saw that twenty-five minutes of the hour-long session had taken place. I had not asked Doris one single question about herself. The only thing she had said so far was "Well, you need to tell it like it is!" I always ask my clients to hold all of their comments until I, at least, share my initial impressions. I then ask if any of what I have been telling them makes sense and what comments they have regarding my initial insights. In this way clients know you have not been fishing for information from them. You have not asked one single question and they have not said a single word during the initial impressions. I have found that this creates a more "power-packed" reading for them.

My initial impressions do not usually take up so much time, so I thought I had better stop and ask Doris if any of this information was making sense to her. She exclaimed that it made complete sense to her and was already extremely helpful for her to hear these things. With a completely open heart, this woman told me that she had spent her entire seventy years trying to be the male that her father had always wanted and even demanded of her to be. Even though her body was female, she was never able to express herself as a female in childhood, and over the years she became more and more uncomfortable as a female. Doris shared her deepest, most intimate pain with me about her life.

Here is a breakdown of all the connections she made and told me about after the first twenty-five minutes of the session:

| My Assessment | Client's Connection |
|---|---|
| Washed out vague violet in the head area. | She has been feeling confused about what is happening physically to her lately. She also could not think clearly and had been feeling very muddled. |

| No energy in the throat and neck area. | She recently had surgery to unclog the carotid arteries on both sides of her neck. |
|---|---|
| Heavy maroon/burgundy shield across her heart. | She felt anger regarding specific situations in her life and named these situations. |
| Daisy opening and closing as if in a breathing pattern. | She had trouble taking in the breath of life. She was a smoker and hoped to quit soon. |
| Pine cone, dry itchy skin. | She has had psoriasis since she was twelve years old. She was completely free of it for a short time but then it came back much worse than it has ever been. |
| Energy deflecting away from her vaginal area or first chakra. | Doris had never felt like a female and connected more with feeling male since she had to take over so many responsibilities for her father who passed away when she was young. She also did not form relationships with people who might become lovers or life partners. She had always struggled with this. |
| Legs were not visible during my initial impressions. | She felt physically depleted in general, but especially felt that her legs could not hold her up. She could not get up the stairs or walk long enough to go to the store due to the weakness. |

Your initial impressions are not only based on your perceptions but also the client's ability to be energetically open and eager to gain insight into their life. On rare occasions, the client seems to be in a "prove it to me" or an argumentative place in life. Try not to involve yourself in the battle because you will not be able to win. You cannot battle your way into a client's energy field because the client never loses control even during these very intimate readings. They are in charge of opening up to the information or closing down to it. It is difficult to change our thinking and our life and to view it from a different angle. You can only let them know how you perceive their struggle and ask that they allow the reading to happen. Doris was, at first, afraid because I was so accurately describing her life-long personal secret. But with an open heart she allowed the reading to continue and she received a gentle healing because of it.

**Practice with Five Case Studies**

Many people learn more deeply and more permanently through

stories and examples of real life experiences. These case studies are real and have been chosen because the people have confirmed the accuracy of the reading. Do not project your energy to these people because I have changed their names to protect their privacy. As each case is discussed, reflect back to all that you have learned and practiced throughout this book and apply each theory to these cases. As I describe the energy, the sensations, and the images regarding each person, you can come to your own conclusions and your own insights.

Practice with the following cases. A summary of each case is presented after the description. Do not read the summary until you write down your own assessment and meaning for each portion of the reading. Then read the summary of each case to compare with your findings. If your findings are different from mine, embrace them and do not dismiss yours. Combine your awareness with my summaries.

Practice. Practice. Practice. Practice.

## Case 1: Susie

I projected my energy field into Susie's head and saw the full spectrum of a rainbow arching inside of her head, completely crossing her head. Each color was clear and bright.

I then noticed that Susie was sending rose-colored beams of light outward toward an angel who was standing behind her. The angel seemed to be filled with white light and stood very close to Susie, their energies intermingled.

Susie's shoulders were tight and the energy was slightly darker throughout the muscles. "Your left shoulder is filled with hot prickly balls like thistles in a field." Scanning downward to her heart revealed a giant yellow daisy. I informed her that her solar plexus, just above the belly button, was also yellow but filled with dark dots that appeared like bullet holes. The word "father" popped into my mind, and I told her that as I described the holes.

I was forcefully drawn down to her second chakra, just below the belly button, and saw tendrils or finger-like fibers all throughout her lower abdomen. The fibers appeared thick in deep brownish red and at the same time the area had a slight orange color.

Write down your assessment of Susie now.

## Susie's Summary

*Head*—It would be significant if one or more of the color spectrum of a rainbow was missing. What if the color yellow was missing? It might tell you that there is a great deal of energy within her brain and head. Was she thinking in details or was she possibly struggling with keeping track of detailed information? Was she feeling disorganized in her life? Remember that the yellow that was present was clear, signifying detailed and organized thinking. It is also significant that the rainbow appeared inside of her head, arching across her entire head, encompassing both sides of her brain.

Her rainbow was deep within her head under the skull, so this might represent that she is able to put Spirit into action in her life and in her thoughts. What would you think if the rainbow was outside and above her head? I might conclude that her seventh chakra center was remarkably active and her energy was extending out and into the spirit realms of awareness. The color bands suggested clear, balanced, and highly attuned positive energy.

*Angel*—Clearly a profound connection was happening for both of them. The angel's energy flooded into Susie's and Susie was radiating energy outward from her crown. Their energy intermingled. Susie was consciously connecting to angelic guidance, and the angel was clearly responding for her.

*Shoulders*—The darker sense of her shoulders signified a tight constriction of energy. She agreed that her left shoulder felt as if it was full of hot needles and she constantly felt pain in both shoulders whenever she was tense about something. Left shoulder problems often mean that the person is taking on too much responsibility, shouldering too much in her own life and possibly too much for someone else. She also felt she was trying to deal with anger about all of her duties.

*Heart*—I told her that her heart was so open and I could tell she was transforming her anger into the positive. Susie shared how she had been going through counseling to work through old issues.

*Solar plexus*—She confirmed that she still had issues with her father's abuse but was working on it. Over the years he had repeatedly shot holes in her self-esteem and her energy field reflected that abuse. The solar plexus is the core of who we are as individuals. When our self-esteem is strong, the energy is strong in that area, not riddled with small holes. She had taken multiple abusive hits from her father.

*Second chakra*—This is the energy center of propagation, the creation of babies, but it is also about the creation of our individuality and our individual life. It was full of angry-looking, tangled threads. Much of Susie's anger was turned back toward herself. She expressed feeling a great deal of self-blame, which interfered and restricted her life. I knew that she had been doing some emotional work through counseling because the slight orange that I saw, while murky, meant the beginning of confidence and self-worth. I could see that she had a terrible case of endometriosis but did not diagnose it. I described only what I perceived. She shared that she was diagnosed with endometriosis and was scheduled for surgery.

## Case 2: Jane

The left side of Jane's head emitted a darker energy than the right side. I felt a dull ache from the left hemisphere of the brain and the ache continued into her jaw. She displayed a small but bright purple light from her third eye and the same from the top of her head. Jane's eyes and ears seemed bright with light shining outward. I paid no attention to her nose and went on to her neck and throat. A small streak of inflamed red was shooting out from the right side of her throat, but the other portions of her neck and throat had a nice warm orange energy.

I did not sense anything noticeable about the shoulders except a vague rosy-pink beginning to appear in my mind. The intensity of the rosy-pink began to build as I assessed Jane's chest and her heart. This same color formed a large spiral outward from her body, and at the same time a smaller spiral of the same shade also spiraled back into her body and heart.

I continued into the abdomen and looked deeply into her gallbladder and then the liver. Both had an even look in some yellows. Nothing else popped into my mind in that area so I looked into Jane's stomach to find more yellows and slight gold. I did not see anything inside of the organ of the stomach. I shifted my gaze to the left side of Jane's abdomen and went deeply into the pancreas and then the spleen. The pancreas felt normal and healthy but the spleen had the sensation of moving slowly and even felt sluggish. I looked down into it and noticed a thickness and a dim energetic color of light brown. When I described her spleen, Jane gasped. I asked her not to tell me anything until I finished the reading.

On inspection of Jane's lower abdomen, I became aware of a line of bubbles rising up from a small section of the lower left quadrant of the abdomen. The base of her spine and groin appeared in warm reds and orange and that energy rose up easily from her right leg. Her left leg had the same energy but slightly diminished. Upon scanning down her left leg, I noticed an even darker shade around her ankle and foot.

Write down your assessment of Jane now.

**Jane's Summary**

*Head*—Jane admitted that she had been stressed and trying to figure out a lot of things lately. I told her that she might be clenching her teeth, but she was not aware of doing that, at least while awake. The small bright purple at the top of her head and at her third eye might show that Jane had recently been using her intuition more and recognizing it. She acknowledged using her instincts and trusting them more. She agreed that she noticed everything around her, thus the increased energy in her eyes and ears.

I did not see anything about her nose during my initial scan, but at the end of the reading she told me she had not been able to smell for over six months. I went back to her nose to examine it more closely and noticed that the right nostril seemed to be shut down but the left nostril had energy flowing in and out of it. When I mentioned this to her, Jane stated that she'd had some sense of smell the last couple of weeks.

*Throat*—I told her that she had a small red streak jutting out from her throat, as is often the case when someone lashes out in anger. She smiled and nodded her head in agreement. She did not hold onto anger but expressed it appropriately, as seen in a red streak shooting outward. Her throat area was a clear orange so I let her know that she expressed herself honestly and clearly.

*Shoulder/Chest*—Jane seemed to handle responsibilities without difficulty because her shoulders seemed even and the energy flowed. The rosy-orange of her upper chest signified that love and confidence had been building in Jane's life. The large spiraling outward and the small spiraling inward showed she gave a great deal of love but struggled to receive love at the same level that she gave. Remember that the inward spiral was smaller than the outward spiral. This made sense to Jane.

*Abdomen*—The yellows might express the confident sense

of self that Jane said she had been feeling lately due to all the counseling, meditating, and yoga she had been doing. The spleen felt sluggish and appeared brown. The organ was thick and dense. Jane told me that six months prior she had her car's upholstery and carpet cleaned. The chemicals overwhelmed her and she immediately lost her sense of smell. Months later it was slowly returning. Now remember that I did not notice anything about her nose, which should have been a clue for me. The fact that I did not notice her nose could have been a signal to me that there was no energy in that area of her face! That should have been a piece of information and not to be overlooked.

*Lower abdomen*—Small bubbles rose up from the lower left section of her abdomen. Jane agreed that she frequently had an uncomfortable pain in the exact spot where the bubbles were. I informed her that there was a leak in her energetic body, which could happen from an emotional trauma or an actual physical trauma. She informed me of a past surgery in that spot.

*Legs*—Jane said that she had greatly increased her exercising routine and had been aware of overdoing it the last couple of weeks. She had multiple aches and pains. Remember, too, that medical intuitives can pick up a stress or struggle in the energy field even before it becomes physical.

**Case 3: Robert**

Robert had multiple issues going on as I entered into his energy field. The left side of his head was clouded over, and in the center of his brain, a line of bubbles rose upward from a dark area. The crown of his head displayed a large, gentle, lovely purple in funnel shape that extended upward for approximately three feet.

He had pain emitting from the right side of his jaw even though the color was good. His throat did not display anything remarkable so I scanned down to the heart center. The shape of a heart like you would see on a valentine card appeared. I looked closely at it and waited. A defined black line zigzagged completely across the valentine heart shape. The edges of the black line were frayed and showed the red of inflammation.

Farther down into the third chakra, the yellowish-orange energy became dim and subdued. I could barely see it. As I scrolled down into his lower abdomen, Robert's lower left side appeared in dark browns. The energy was stagnant, without any flow. The first chakra had the most energetic color in red. I struggled to feel or visualize energy in his legs, but looking more deeply I could find some vague green. His feet were completely dark, with pain releasing from the arch of his right foot.

Spirit guided me to ask Robert to turn around so I could view his backside more clearly. I focused my energetic laser beam into his spine and slowly scanned up and down. All seemed well until I looked into his mid-back. There I saw a dark, blackish, thick spot. I asked my guide to tell me what vertebrae it was seeing. The thought jumped into my mind: T4. The energy was diminished from T4 all the way up his spine toward his head. The energy beneath T4 flowed more naturally.

Write down your assessment of Robert now.

## Robert's Summary

*Head*—The dark energy is stress and some depression. Robert said that he ruminated over and over about a failed relationship and could not seem to get over it. He also remembered he had hit his head on a beam in the same area where the leak appeared. I told him that the large purple emanating from the crown of his head signified an important and valued connection with God or however he sensed a spiritual life. He told me that he had been meditating daily and also prayed throughout the day. I told him that this was all very real and I could tell that he was a devoted meditator by the clear purples rising from his crown chakra.

*Heart*—You might have already surmised that the valentine image of his heart signified a broken heart and the edges were still raw with emotion. We discussed ways to begin the repair of his broken heart, and I warned him that if he continued to ruminate in this way it could become a physical situation that could lead to complications in the physical organ of his heart. (More on healing later.)

*Third Chakra*—Robert had really taken a hit regarding the loss of the relationship. His self-esteem was next to nothing. He was taking on a great deal of the responsibility and was tearing himself up about it. He was racked with dread and guilt, which in turn stifled and constricted the solar plexus, resulting in a barely discernible sense of self.

*Lower abdomen*—The dark brown sluggish area was in the colon. Robert agreed that he had been horribly constipated to the point of feeling ill. I told him that the constipation was in direct correlation to his grief about the woman. "You are literally holding onto old emotional crap, not learning from it and letting it go." When I mentioned this, he realized that he had never been constipated before the breakup and that it did begin a few weeks after his breakup.

*Legs/Feet*—I described the low energy in his legs. Robert told me that he was a truck driver and suffered from aching legs after long distance hauls. He had already noticed pain in the arch of his right foot, and I suggested getting orthotics to give him more support when he gets out of the truck. I suggested elastic stockings and encouraged him to do some muscle tightening exercises while he drove to increase the blood flow. I stressed to him that his body was craving movement. I asked him to walk more when he was at home and not on the road.

*Spine*—Did you notice that the blockage at T4 is directly in line with Robert's broken heart? The two seemed to be linked and again signify the severity of his grief. According to Louise Hay in her book *Heal Your Body*, the T4 vertebrae has the tendency to be affected by bitterness and condemnation. While Robert took much of the responsibility for the failed relationship, he also blamed. The blockage within the spine signifies the severity of his heart break.


## Case 4: Sam

Sam's physical body was greatly overweight and as he walked into my office, he struggled to breathe. When we sat down together I struggled to get into his energy field. I saw a gray, heavy, gelatinous substance completely draping his body. I pushed through it and found that it was formed of multiple layers. I felt a great amount of pressure as I got closer to his physical body. It felt as if the pressure was building up inside of my own body and especially my own head. Sam's head was releasing hot, needle-type forms from the left side of his brain. In spite of all this, the energy of his third eye appeared in light purple.

The heaviness was even thicker over his heart. I suddenly saw six tiny stick figures. Each stick figure was connected by hot, dark maroon-red lines that formed a tangled pattern resembling lace all around his heart. Inside this red ring and closer to his heart was a light green vibration.

I continued to push through the thick, gelatinous vibration throughout the remainder of his body but did not really notice anything remarkable until I scanned into the second chakra. Here I saw six corkscrew forms of springy energy going in all directions and again, all tangled up together. They appeared in that same maroon-red.

His knees were misshapen. The energy field around them was not aligned and they did not look equal. The right knee had four holes piercing through it and pain floating out from the holes in the shape of thin threads. The left knee appeared completely different. It looked as if it was on fire and was larger than the other knee. His left ankle had the same fiery energy as the left knee.

Write down your assessment of Sam now.

## Sam's Summary

*Entire Body*—The gray, layered, gelatinous substance formed a solid protection around Sam. As the protection continued over the years, it became a barrier of sorts, the gray color expressing depression and hopelessness. The layers signify one negative experience after another building up over time. The gelatinous form looked and felt like adipose tissue (fat) that his body physically held. It was as if this man had fat in his energy field and fat in his body. This insulation created a wall between him and the rest of the world. I could not see any energy transference through it as a healthy person would normally have.

*Head*—Sam explained he was feeling more and more depressed and cut off from life. When I described the extreme internal pressure that I was feeling, he said he was diagnosed with uncontrollable high blood pressure. He confirmed that he always had headaches, primarily on the left side of his head. I told him that he had a light purple in the area of his third eye, which signified to me that he had potential to be intuitive, but the small shape and its dim vibration told me he did not put it to use. Sam agreed with that assessment.

*Heart*—I described the strange image within his heart center showing tangles of anger involving six distinct people. The surprised look on his face told me that he definitely recognized what I was talking about. He went into detail about how angry he gets with six family members and how he tries to help them all by giving lots of advice, but no one does what he wants them to do and it angers him. We discussed at length how this pattern of involvement was now at a detrimental level to his body, and I offered some alternative ways to show love and caring to these important people in his life.

I reinforced the fact that the way he was trying to help his family had not changed anything for them and suggested he try some different methods. I also tried to give him hope that the light green energy within the tangled ring told me that he was already bringing in new healing energy into the situation and if he followed through, he would feel emotionally and physically better.

*Second chakra*—Again the six people appeared as six tangled energy springs coiling around each other in a complicated mess. I pointed out that each person carried their own responsibility in this family, but he was also responsible for at least a portion of the stressful anger. I told him that the second chakra is about creation of our own life experiences. He said the reading was making a great deal of sense to him and was very helpful.

*Knees*—Sam confirmed my visions and sensations of his knees. The right knee usually had sharp stabbing pain surging through it, and the left knee was inflamed and full of fluid. My description corresponded with the physician's diagnosis. Sam had been putting off surgery on both knees. The right knee, with four holes and stabbing pain, was bone on bone and required a knee replacement. The left knee, inflamed with a fiery energy, needed steroid injections to calm the inflammation. Knees are about flexibility or rigidity in life. This too corresponded to the six people in his life.

**Case 5: Tammy**

I immediately envisioned a spirit guide standing behind and floating above this middle-aged woman. The female guide smiled down at Tammy and then looked at me with a smile. I smiled back and sent her vibrations of love and appreciation. I told Tammy of her guide's presence and told her that this guide said she sends a blessing to her today. While I had no idea if Tammy believed in spirit guides or not, I informed her regardless of her religion.

Tammy's crown center was actually shaped as a lively green crown and on her forehead was a shiny star. Her throat, although not dark, was simply void of energy. Her heart center appeared as if it had multiple small fires, but the fires felt positive as I viewed them. Hovering above her heart and to the left was a huge ball of vibrant pink energy. The energy was about the size of a basketball.

Her upper abdomen appeared as an enormous flower in full bloom. I blinked a couple of times because I saw a honey bee whirring about the flower, pollinating it. Tammy's lower abdomen pulsated in deep orange, but I quickly observed there seemed to be three separate and distinct energy centers instead of the usual one. The color was good and strong and each spherical center seemed to be circling in a clockwise direction.

Then I had to blink again because I saw the form of a human male at the base of her spine. I looked more closely and asked him to show himself to me and to show me why he was there. I saw him brighten with more light and he sent a wave of love to me and to Tammy.

Her legs were low in energy but showed a medium green color. Pain emanated from the inside of her right leg just above her ankle. That same pain was also shooting out from the bottom of her right foot. Both feet appeared in a dull, dim green.

Write down your assessment of Tammy now.

## Tammy's Summary

*Spirit guide*—We have different types of guides for different reasons and at different times in our lives. This guide was of a high order. She was strong and hovered way above the floor. She was vibrating in such a way that it seemed she could not even touch the material ground.

*Head*—An energetic crown in Tammy's crown chakra represented an advanced level of development with Spirit. The light green color sent a signal of its newer development. It symbolized Tammy's more recent spiritual awareness. A star in the third eye told me she was cognizant of receiving universal information and was incorporating that intuitive intelligence into her current life.

*Heart*—The small fires felt positive and seemed to be burning away the old negativity. This positive perception leaped into my mind, so I trusted it and informed Tammy. I was also delighted to tell her that the huge ball of pink energy is love or a lover attempting to enter into her life. Things coming into someone's life seem to show up on our left, the receiving side of the body. Since the energy ball hung in the air about three to four feet away, the distance revealed that the love had not manifested directly in life or the person was not willing to allow new love to happen. Because of its vibrant energy, it would certainly be a positive addition in her life. She stated she felt a partner was just out of her reach. We explored her ability to receive in life and how she might be getting in her own way.

*Abdomen/Second chakra*—The full bloom of her abdomen revealed the strong sense of self that Tammy said she had felt lately. The surprise appearance of a bee suggested she was actively pollinating her individual creativity. She shared examples of how she was breaking out into her own and felt alive for the first time.

The three spinning whirlwind shapes in her second chakra, however, revealed some struggles. I told her I had not seen this before. I asked her if she had so many things going in her life and so many different interests that she did not know which way to go. Tammy heartily agreed and said that the world offered so many opportunities and ideas that she did not know which way to go first. I suggested an assignment to assist her in organizing her energetic matrix first, which in turn would bring more balance in her body and in her life.

*First chakra*—I do not usually visualize the form of a man in someone's chakra so when this or something else unusual happens, I begin by asking specific questions and "listening" for the answers. In this case, the male form felt and looked positive. I informed Tammy that she was receiving many symbols and messages in this reading that a new relationship was available to her if she chose it. She thought she already knew who the man might be.

*Legs/feet*—Tammy admitted that she had not been physically moving her body and sometimes she even forgets about having legs. She agreed that she sometimes felt a sharp pain in her leg as I had described it. I told her that her body was telling her to walk more, and in fact her body seemed to be yearning for movement. She felt that same sensation but often ignored it.

These five case studies have been another opportunity to apply what you have been learning and to put medical intuition into action. Accept your own intuitive insights as important and incorporate them into your own development. To excel as a medical intuitive, you must experience each and every instinct and you must honor each and every insight that pops into your mind from the cosmos.

Let yourself recognize and feel positive about the progress you have already made. Take a moment to remember the advancements you have made from each experience in this course. Your instincts and abilities have accelerated. Allow yourself to acknowledge your growing awareness.

# Chapter Eleven

## The Professional Medical Intuitive

### Valuable Keys for the Professional Medical Intuitive

Let's bring this journey together with a quick review of all that you have done.

1. We began with a discussion about medical intuition, including what it is and who is already doing it. Most people, including healing practitioners, have no idea that they are receiving vital intuitive information. For example, massage therapists, physical therapists, nurses, physicians, energy workers, lightworkers, and people without any medical background naturally pick up intuitive information about others. It is not a mystical gift. We are naturally wired to receive intuitive information on a minute-by-minute basis.

2. We discussed the history of medical intuition and that it was first documented in the 1840s by a physician. In fact, medical intuition goes back to the beginning of human life on earth. Shamans, herbalists, and healers are pictured in cave drawings before written language was developed. Medical intuition has been a healing modality for centuries. Hearing and understanding the source of their illness helps people open their eyes to a deeper and more significant level of awareness and healing.

3. The electrical nature of the mind, the body, the earth, and the Universe was described and discussed. Physicians order electrically based tests because the human body is an electrically based entity. We receive EEGs to document the

electrical movement throughout the brain. EKGs monitor the electrical movement throughout the heart, and EMGs measure the electrical current throughout muscles. We see the electrical defibrillator paddles being used on TV when a heart stops. The jolt of electricity often restarts a heart because each beat of the heart begins with an electrical spark. According to the HeartMath Institute, the heart even has brain cells and personal conscious memory.

4.  Information has energy and energy has information. We are simply learning to tap into those living systems to access intuitive information. One of your initial awareness assignments was to notice each person in your life as soul energy before noticing the body or the personality. Remember what you discovered?

Each individual has a story and that unceasing story is created, generated, and influenced not only by our thoughts and subsequent emotions, but also by choices and decisions, genetic heritage, energy patterns of our ancestors, upbringing, parents' lifestyle, food and nutrition, relationships, Earth's electromagnetic field, current life experiences, current life history, past lives, and the intergalactic realm. Any of these influences may spontaneously enter your medical intuition reading because you are entering the dynamic personal story of each human. A portion of that story is contained in the physical brain, but the entire story, in epic proportions, resides in the eternal mind or soul of each individual. The aura is the energy of the soul and the soul is the never-ending saga of development. Medical intuition accesses the Divine and it accesses the struggles of the human experience. Illness comes in various degrees of severity and each ailment, from a stubbed toe to a fatal illness, is the body signaling us. Each signal contains a world of information, a chapter in the saga.

5. Ethical issues of confidentiality for others and respect for the intimate information that you are entering into were reviewed. Remember, as you go out into the world as a medical intuitive, you cannot diagnosis unless you have a medical degree. You can, however, describe the look, the feel, the layers of emotions, and the history involved within an illness. Asking permission has been emphasized over and over again. I agree we can do no harm sending love and healing to someone in need. My point in asking for permission is to involve the receiver in the process. When someone verbally or psychically gives us permission to enter into their story, they more actively participate in their own process.

6. Remember that if you think you cannot do medical intuition or any other type of intuition, you will never be able to do it. We cannot go where our thoughts do not go. Think and know you are picking up information from the cosmos and information from the human body. Talk about your medical intuitive work with pride and do not hide it. You are an invaluable asset for people who are struggling and have no idea how to heal.

7. Remember that our heads, our brains, and our bodies are one unit. What happens in our mind must happen in our body, positively and negatively. Fear, emotion, and expectations are restrictive, resistant emotions that block the currents of your energy, your instincts, and your intuition. You are not the only one who feels fear. Your clients are afraid of what you will find in their bodies and in their stories. Be kind and sensitive.

8. Imagination is the energy of spirit and the energy of intuition. It will always feel as if you are dreaming it all up. You are not making it up. Intuition is real. Notice your imagination and let it flow. Daydream with purpose and daydream deliberately to access the spirit mind.

9. Intent is a deliberate, laser-like focus, and your focus is power packed. Use it wisely with the highest, most divine purpose. Human intent can move mountains and create natural miracles. We humans are a tremendously powerful link in the system of the cosmos. We are not meant to be the weakest link. This is the greatest lesson to learn in our lifetime.

   Remember the steps of setting intent? Remember that it is not about trying harder. Intuition is the ability to receive information. It is not about working harder.

10. Have you been meditating? If not, get started with only two minutes each day. Go back to Meditation Made Simple in Chapter Four and put it into action. As your mind calms, your energy body will glow in a lighter, finer frequency. Build it up and feel the love with the section entitled Enrich Your Light Body, also in Chapter Four.

11. Building up your electrical frequencies prepares you to invite divine intelligence and to receive its guidance. Have you been dialoging daily with your spirit guide specialist? Your guide will rock your world and sooth your soul all at the same time. Your guides will direct and enhance your intuitive insights if you call them. You do not need to work alone as a medical intuitive. Your specialist is there for you if you allow them to participate in your work and in your life. Remember . . . you are the powerful link in the system.

12. Remember that intuitives use the term "seeing" in a very general way. In the intuitive world, seeing really means the following:

    • Thoughts that pop into your mind.

    • Symbols in your mind's eye that represent a volume of information.

    • Pictures unfolding entire scenes in front of you.

    • Body sensations that are not your own.

- Sounds in another's energy field.

- Sensing unusual smells.

- Spirit directing your focus.

- Honoring the "knowing" that flows through you.

13. You are in charge of you and in charge of your energy field. Take control of it as you take control of your own thought processes. Direct your energy field like stretching an elastic band or pulling warm taffy across a room. Go to Playful Steps to Direct Your Energy in Chapter Five for a reminder. This is your laser beam. Here is why you are becoming more and more accurate. Your laser beam is the ultimate key for excellence.

14. Where is the mind's eye and how do you work with it? You stared at an object in the space around you until it imprinted in your mind. You then closed your eyes and noticed where and how the image appeared for you. You then saw the image of a tree and learned that the precision of a medical intuitive is noticing every single detail of the color, the symbol, and the client's story.

15. The aura, like noticing every detail about the symbol of the tree, has many characteristics that give the medical intuitive an in-depth description of the person you are working with. We also began to put medical intuition into practice with a self-scan.

    How are you different now? Just notice—the aura is surging with information and has been affected by so many situations and circumstances. It is the accumulation of all that you have been, all that you are now, and all that is possible in the future. The Color Interpretation of the Aura in Chapter Seven can be copied and used as a quick reference for you.

16. The chakras are generators creating vital energy. They are also centers of information regarding primary life issues

that we all struggle with. Do you remember the main issues associated with each chakra and the connection between the struggle and the vibration of the chakras? Review them to refresh yourself with the details they provide you with. Are you aware of your own inner chakras? Consider completing a self-scan of your entire auric field and complete a chakra assessment before moving forward. It might seem different now as you progress in your medical intuitive discoveries.

17. Remember that the right or left side of the body is often a key detail to notice pertinent information affecting your client. While you do not need to take a college course in anatomy and physiology, you do need to know where all the primary body parts are and what side of the body the internal organs are located. For instance, can you quickly identify where the liver is or what part of the body the gallbladder occupies?

18. Take the time to learn the emotional component that is associated with each organ and each portion of the body. It is vital that you understand how the body responds to thought and emotion and the effect it has on the human body. We looked at the possible influence that past lives have on our current bodies. Be prepared to see unusual images of times long ago. Remember, even if you do not believe in reincarnation your clients might believe. Utilize the beliefs and awareness of your clients. Even if you or your client do not believe in past lives, utilize it as a story, jam-packed full of significant intuitive information for your client. Look at the action or non-action of the event showing itself to you and go from there. In other words, do not dismiss it as fantasy.

19. Remember the strange, the weird, and the wild? Well, there is more of that as you progress in your medical intuition consultations. The more people that you assist, the more you will come across wondrous uncharted realms that

will open your inner knowing. Be excited and explore these worlds. Keep your light body at a high frequency by maintaining a large, expanded, bright, shimmery, clear auric field.

20. The more you take action as a medical intuitive, the more you will feel the flow and understand all the associations you are providing for the person before you. We must always know with certainty that the reading we provide will be remarkable for the person who sits before us. This is their special, exciting time to hear and learn about themselves. You are participating in a special intimate relationship with another human. Make each moment with every person special and also positive in some way.

21. Do not carry the burdens of others and do not take those burdens home with you. Allow every person to have their own path and their own choices. Each second of every day contains a myriad of choice for each of us. Have you noticed that you cannot make anyone change, even your own loved ones? You can offer the information that you are picking up, but you must then release the outcome. It is not yours to bear and never was. This is the largest struggle for the medical intuitive, and it is one of the most important lessons in the physical world.

**Creating Your Own Patterns**

I have altered the pattern of my sessions a few times over the years. I used to ramble on for half an hour before I stopped to take a breath or ask the client for their response regarding all I had shared with them. I had given them so much information, so fast and so surprisingly intimate, that people could not remember most of the details and could barely respond. I had to remind them of my intuitive insights because they were so overwhelmed. It was a blast of information and too much for a person to take in, let alone assimilate and respond to.

In the beginning, I would also allow an individual to tell me all their physical ailments, diseases, and struggles before we entered into the reading. I found, time and again, that I did not have as much credibility regarding the intuitive information I had for them. They made comments such as "Well, I just mentioned that to you." People, especially if they hear information that is difficult or emotional, will at first go into denial or rejection. If they think you are fishing for information, they will always discredit it and subsequently decide that you just made it all up anyway. There is a fine line to follow that will allow the most optimal situation for the person you are reading for.

Here is a general pattern for a medical intuitive reading:

1. Greet the person on the phone, Skype, or in person.

2. Immediately inform them that you do not want them to disclose any information about their medical situation until later in the session. Tell the client that you want to tell them your initial impressions before they offer any information. They will be delighted.

3. Inform them that their job during the session is to feel open, excited, and fascinated about this special time that they have given themselves.

4. If you decide to record your sessions, then start recording at this point. You might decide to use the human body form to draw and write on or you might record the sessions instead. If you use a form, document as you undergo the session because it is difficult to remember all that rushes in.

5. Ask for a quiet moment together to connect in with each other. Between thirty seconds to one minute is usually long enough, but take more if you need it. If it goes much longer your client will wonder what is going on.

6. Watch the clock occasionally and give your initial impressions. Even if you are on a roll, do not go over ten minutes or so because it is too much for most people.

7.  Never ask the client any questions. They will be convinced that you are searching for information rather than using your intuition. The only question you might ask is "Does this make any sense to you?" I do remind them to not tell me anything about their medical condition or their struggles yet.

8.  At the end of the scanning assessment, ask if there is any area of their body that they would like you to examine more deeply. Remind them not to tell you why they want you to look more closely.

9.  Ask what specific questions they have. As they ask questions, watch their energy field, for it will alter as they speak, giving you even more information.

10. Inform them when the time is about to end. Ask if any questions still linger.

11. In order to turn the responsibility for their health back to them, give them an assignment. I literally call it a homework assignment. (More on this later.) I also ask them to listen to the recording many times, for it will assist them to stay on track for their own healing awareness.

12. Finalize the payment for your assessment.

The goals for this pattern are threefold:

1.  To not overwhelm the person with more information than they can assimilate.

2.  To encourage credibility for yourself but especially credibility of the healing information that you are giving them. You do not want them to discount this valuable information because they decided that you probed for the facts before you gave the reading.

3.  To turn the focus and responsibility for their health back to their own abilities by giving the individual a homework assignment.

I record many of my sessions because people simply cannot remember all the tiny details that are brought forth in a reading. You can purchase a digital recorder, download the recording to your computer and burn it to a CD, or email the recording to them. I find that most people prefer to receive the recorded session through their email.

Feel free to use the pattern that I have described above. You may find yourself following my pattern and slowly altering it as your confidence grows. It is time to experiment in creating your own session patterns that will fit your needs and the needs of your clients.

**What to Do When You Miss a Diagnosed Illness**

I just finished a phone session with an older man with a soft, gentle voice when his wife instantly got on the phone and screamed in a scary, husky voice, "You didn't say a word about his brain tumor!"

I loudly replied, "Stop right there and do not tell me another thing!" I was surprised at her silence. "I did miss it but give me a moment to check his head again." We were all on a speaker phone so I asked the man for permission to go back into his head. When he said yes, I deliberately sent a very specific laser beam focus deep into his head and repeated his name silently in my own mind. (Repeating the person's name will work for you in a target-like manner to increase the aim of the focused intent.)

**Essential Point:**
*Repeat the person's name to enhance a targeted,*
*focused intent.*

Like a CAT scan, I went back and forth across each hemisphere of his brain. I was viewing his brain in thin segments, each segment an inch-thick slice. "The tumor is in the right hemisphere of your brain. It is approximately three inches down from the top of your head and about 1½ inches in from the right side of your skull at about ear level. It is round with a thin transparent membrane and it is fluid filled.

"Since you already have a diagnosis I will share with you that I am picking up that you are not in danger from this tumor. It is, however, developing because of a resistance to taking some action, a resistance in creativity, a resistance to becoming someone you already are—"

His wife yelled again, "That's exactly what the doctors said it looked like!"

Whew. I was relieved. His wife went on to say that she had been after him to work with his art more than he does.

I piped in, "Well, sir, that may be what I was referring to earlier when I said the transparent tumor is a resistance to something." He quietly agreed. Together we all worked through it and closed the session calmly.

### Essential Point:
*Don't be alarmed when you miss something.*

I offer you this painful example in order for you to learn from my experience. You will miss things, and you will miss things that are important to the client. I also know that we will miss the things that are not really important according to our guide specialists. When the client feels I have missed something, I firmly tell the client that it did not come up because the guides did not think it important or they did not want to delve into it at this time. When that happens, and it probably will, stop the person if you possibly can, and ask for a moment to look more closely at a specific area of their body.

Don't be alarmed when you miss something that the person knows they have. The session is still not about you. Refocus on the client. If your focus shifts to you and your error, you will not be able to recover the clarity of your soul mind. No matter what happens during a reading, do not make it about yourself in any way. Instead, create a powerful laser beam of focused intent and go deeply into the section of the person's body. Give them whatever you get in a kind tone of voice, but do not dwell on or apologize for missing something. As you dialog with them, focus and point out the added information that you receive for them.

## How to Create Healing with Medical Intuition

Many little cone-shaped vortexes swirled in every direction from Connie's head. Each cone was about the same size and without any evident color vibration. Her head felt and looked balanced in greens. There was a gray thickness around her neck with a few red, hot lines projecting outward from the gray.

I said, "You are trying to hold down a great deal of emotion, but every once in a while anger shoots out and then you go back to quiet." As I described these impressions, a protective shield came across my vision, coming from the right and the left equally. The shield came close, blocking out my vision of her completely. I asked her in a calm, soothing voice to relax and be fascinated with our time together. The shield fell away and I could see her energy again.

A dark emotional energy draped over her left shoulder and hung down over her heart. I watched and quickly noticed that my own heart felt very heavy in my chest. I actually felt something pressing down against my heart. As the pressing continued, a long achiness rose up from the organ of her heart. I informed Connie of this feeling within my own body but assured her that I was not taking it on or making it my own. I only wanted her to know what I was sensing for her. She nodded that she understood and verbally agreed with my assessment up to this point.

I continued scanning Connie's internal organs in her abdomen, but the sensations of her heart kept pulling my attention back to it again and again. When I mentioned this, the wall slid back across her and stood between us. She disappeared again. We stopped the reading and I told her how the screen was blocking our ability to continue. I told her what I was sensing and how it appeared. She told me that I was correct about the protection I sensed. She stated that she felt herself blocking me out and was aware of it both times when I mentioned it, saying, "I just do not want to look at some things in my life."

When she said it was all right to go on, I told her that there seemed to be three components to her heartache. First, I saw a dead man stretched out on the floor. "That was my uncle," she responded. I continued telling her that another human form was showing itself, but this human was headless. I stated that this person had dementia or Alzheimer's disease and felt as if they no longer had a head or a brain. "That was my grandmother," she said calmly. "She got so she didn't know anything or anyone."

I continued trying to see the third element of her heartache, but I finally had to tell Connie that I simply could not see it because she would not allow herself to see or feel it. She blurted out, "I have had many miscarriages." I asked her to allow me to look into her lower abdomen and discovered a large yellow flower with big open petals, but it had an empty hole where the center should be.

Connie then asked me to look at her ovaries and fallopian tubes. The left ovary and tube appeared dark and quiet with no activity but the right one was bright in yellow and orange. She stated that the medical tests confirmed what I saw energetically. The physicians told her that the left ovary was not producing but the right one seemed to be functioning.

I returned to the image of the empty center of the flower that sat in the very center of her second chakra between the two ovaries. "It is this flower with the empty center that concerns me and the energy leak in your etheric field. That should not be there."

Connie responded, "I feel so much embarrassment about these miscarriages."

I gently told her that embarrassment is about hiding shame. "Shame is one of the heaviest and most impenetrable energy frequencies. Your shame is adding to the obstruction and is showing up as emptiness in the center of a flower in full bloom. The emptiness is increasing because of the shame and the leak. The open petals tell me that having a baby is possible for you, but you must change your focus toward carrying a baby to full term and stop thinking of your failures in this manner. It is imperative that you transform shame into a more positive feeling, and we need to close the leak."

Connie followed my instructions and together we began sending healing to the leak to close it up. After a few moments, I told her that I saw a Band-Aid placed over the leak. Connie exclaimed excitedly, "I was imagining a Band-Aid over it because that is what you do when there is an opening that needs to heal!" We both giggled. I told her that this energy work is very real and that is why I could see her Band-Aid.

"Now you need to fill the center of that flower and fire it up!" I asked Connie to imagine a very warm orange color filling up her lower abdomen and to imagine the feel of it from her front to her back, through the thickness of her body. "Imagine it fired up, full of life." I asked her to imagine both of her ovaries fired up as well.

I watched her energy field as she did what I asked of her. At first nothing happened, but slowly I witnessed a dim orange beginning to build up. Even though I was focusing on orange, I began to see pink swirling into the orange. I told her that Spirit was bringing in pink of self-love and asked Connie to include orange and pink together. Both energies began to build more strength as she practiced there with me.

I then asked her to feel fire in her lower abdomen and let her body give her a physical sensation of fire. I could see the energy increase a little more. I then asked her to feel pink love in that same area and let her body show her the sensations of pink filling her. Connie's abdomen came alive. I told her how successful she was because I could see it happening. She was taking more control of her energy field and creating a finer frequency within her own body.

Most societies think intuitives have magical powers. While it does seem magical and it feels magical in nature, the clients are ultimately in control of their energy field, consciously or unconsciously. We are in charge of what we assimilate or what deflects from our minds and bodies. In short, we cannot force anyone to heal no matter how strongly we work for them and no matter how strongly we care. You must remember that each person's life is completely up to them. You can only give to them when they ask and release them onto their own journey when they go.

Medical intuition is based on a natural and powerful sensing mechanism that is built into our body. We all have this mechanism. We can improve its function, block it, or ignore it completely. It is natural to know these things about our self, about each other, and for each other. Notice the flow of the scan for Doris that was described earlier. Doris was open and willing to allow the information to be assessed, and she was willing and open to make changes based on the information that she received.

William A. Tiller, PhD, professor emeritus at Stanford University, is famous for his research regarding the human mind and the power of intention. He describes in his paper "Subtle Energy Actions and Physical Domain Correlations: Consciousness, Intentionality and Subtle Energies" the following: "The body's electric and magnetic fields provide the necessary conditions for homeostasis at the chemical level. Detection of imbalances at the electric/magnetic field levels would be an early warning factor of coming potential disruptions in the chemical homeostasis condition, and which, if unchecked, would eventually result in repercussions at the body's functional level. Research and study of hypnosis and hypnotic effects revealed that the human body can exhibit truly remarkable feats of strength and endurance— attesting to an important linkage of body/mind, in which the mind can influence not only the body's structure and function, but also its chemistry and electric/magnetic fields."

The medical intuitive is able to discern an imbalance or an illness when it has manifested physically, but we can also sense a potential illness before it manifests. We pick up very subtle signals in the energy field that medical tests such as MRIs, CAT scans, or x-rays cannot find. The illness will not show up in these medical tests because the illness has not yet formed enough density to show any physical evidence. Illness happens somewhere in the energy field first. The energy signature begins in the electromagnetic matrix around the human body, and as it builds energy, it develops more substance and eventually manifests on a physical level. The medical intuitive feels, sees, or experiences an alteration in the energy field before it manifests.

Go back and review Tony's situation in the section titled Medical Intuition as a Healing Technique in Chapter One. You will notice that Tony did not have a physical illness presenting at the time of his session. He was perplexed about his anxiety and had been curtailing his emotions that led to a restriction in his heart center. That restriction could possibly have resulted in a heart or lung condition or illness if it had continued. His medical intuition session created a healing opportunity for him to heal a situation before it became an illness.

Healing can also take place for a person whose illness has developed further and has actually manifested in the physical body. One must be vigilant in this case to describe only your perceptions and insights so you do not inadvertently give a medical diagnosis. If you see a tumor, for example, you must describe it but not say the word "tumor." Unless you are a licensed physician, you cannot offer a specific name to what you perceive.

### Essential Point:
*Cancer does not mean the end of physical life.*

In the initial few moments of meeting Anita, I did not pick up her history of cancer, nor did I sense that she was currently diagnosed with cancer. She revealed a beautiful shade of green equally in both hemispheres of her brain. A ring or cloud of thicker red hovered in the air around her head. I told her that she had been working on herself and it had a dramatic positive effect because the healing energy of green was literally pushing away the old negative thought patterns. I told her that the ring of thick red was still hanging in the air around her. "It does not appear within your head but is floating outside of your head and beginning to dissolve. Whatever you are doing, keep it up." I did not know about the cancer until the end of her session.

Spiky, hot needles shot out from her left shoulder and some tightness pulled the muscles from her neck down to that shoulder. I said something was injuring that shoulder and she admitted that she always carries her briefcase on that shoulder but was not aware of any problem or pain in that shoulder. I told her that a medical intuitive often picks up struggles before they manifest physically. I suggested a briefcase on wheels.

Anita's heart appeared in that same green as the energy in her head, but looking farther down into her heart I suddenly saw an intricate pattern like lace weaving all around inside of it. "You are a very complicated and multifaceted person. I see an intricate lace pattern inside of your heart, but it is not a tangled mess as I have seen with others. It is a beautiful pattern. Spirit tells me that there were many tangles in the past, but because of all the internal work you have done, you have transformed many emotional experiences into lace. Whatever you are doing, you must keep it up." I still did not sense that she had cancer.

Her solar plexus appeared clear and bright. In fact, the more I shared my observations, the brighter her entire energy field became. As the light inside of her physical body continued to shine, I also observed a dark energy, approximately the same size of her torso, hanging in the air approximately a foot away. The dark energy did not touch her body but floated in the air nearby as if her shadow was detached from her. "You are having a full-bodied release of old heaviness and old guck. I must tell you that I do not even know why I am saying the phrase 'full-bodied release,' but that is what I am hearing."

Her gallbladder and liver seemed normal and so did her pancreas and spleen on her left side. I was having trouble sensing her kidneys, so I asked her if I could place my hands on her back at the level of her kidneys. The energy on the right side fluctuated so rapidly that I could not get a fix on it and I was having trouble even describing the movement that I saw. I told Anita that I had never visualized this formation and movement before, but I tried to describe it anyway. The left kidney seemed normal with some brightness but not the frantic movement and fluctuations as the right side. The left kidney released small sharp pain and in another moment a little more pain shot outward. I informed her that I felt needles releasing when there was stress in the area.

Anita then told me that her right kidney was removed fifteen years ago because of cancer. "That explains why I was seeing such random movement and energetic disorganization. There is no organ to give the energy a foundation to work with." When I have had the opportunity to work with an amputee, the energy often appears in a similar manner, but not always.

Her colon's energy contained a hot red line of inflammation running along its length. Anita said that the inflammation concurred with a medical diagnosis of a fistula that she had recently received. Anita's first chakra and groin area seemed to have transparent filaments rising into the center of the lower abdomen. They resembled fine black lines, like a pencil sketch of a tree with only a few branches. I told her that this was not normal and she needed to have it checked by a physician. She confirmed what I already knew. She had been diagnosed with cancer of the bladder.

I maintained my professional demeanor and told her it was important to know that the cancer did not appear very solid, and in fact seemed like a few thin, wispy branches of a willow tree. "Cancer usually appears to me like heavy black shiny tar, similar to hot asphalt being poured on a road. I really want you to understand that this is a very good sign. It does not look developed or dense as I always see cancer, and it is not even as fibrous like I see endometriosis. The formation of this, in fact, is more transparent and fragile. It does not look or feel durable like other cancers that I have seen." Once again, I restated, "Whatever you are doing, keep it up because it is working for you."

We talked about creating a healing energy exercise to do and she was eager to do it. I became quiet and asked my spirit specialist for direction. "I am told that you are to place your hands at the base of this filament tree, which is literally on your groin. So place your hands on your groin, which is also the urethra, and send the most beautiful color upward." Anita stopped me and said she usually runs her energy downward. I checked again with my specialist and was told to have her push energy from her hands upward and to choose a color that was beautiful to her.

She immediately said turquoise and began to practice. I could see a slight movement in her bladder but before I could tell her, Anita said that she was changing the color to yellow like the sun. I saw the energy brighten somewhat but not significantly. Again, before I could mention there was not much movement yet, she announced, "No, it needs to be gold!" Anita's first and second chakra promptly burst into golden vibrations.

"Now that is the correct energy!" I announced and told her why. I encouraged her to feel the gold energy as she also imagined it and saw it.

What a beautiful, remarkable, and intimate process I was able to share with Anita. She was far from death. In fact, she was more vital than most people coming into my office, and she was excited to participate in her healing. It is never too late to encourage healing, no matter the severity of the illness you are witnessing. This is the point where miracles take place. When there is no hope, we can give hope. When we assist in giving a sick person a new way of thinking or a new understanding of their situation, a healing takes place. Healing is not always the opposite of death. If we can positively assist someone in their death transition, a healing has happened even then.

**Essential Point:**
*Healing is not always the opposite of death.*

I do everything I can to give the power back to each person that I meet with. Once again Esther Hicks seems to describe it so succinctly (from a workshop in San Francisco, California, July 30, 2005): "True healers know that wellness is the order of the day, so they do not allow themselves, even for a moment, to see anything other than that. So, the power of the healer is in the power to influence the one who needs to be healed into a vibration that allows the healing that they are summoning (that they *could* get, even without the healer, but they can get faster with a healer's influence)."

I believe that all healing is eventually self-healing. At the same time, it seems that this world works better when we allow and receive assistance from others. We are not self-contained islands. We do need each other. Even a hermit comes out once in a while to buy groceries. However, as we need each other for support in so many ways, we are ultimately responsible for ourselves and our individual life. When I examined the healing aspect of my medical intuition sessions, I discovered that the sessions had certain elements.

### Six Components of Healing

1. Accurately describe the appearance and the sensations of the area of disease.

2. See and especially feel each person in their healthiest and most vital state of being, however ill they are in the present moment.

3. Create a specific energetic experience that begins an energetic alteration toward healing. The experience includes thinking, feeling, and visualizing in a certain manner.

4. Inform each person how to put the energy assignment into action.

5. Practice the energy assignment immediately during the session and watch their energetic field and their body as they apply the technique. Inform each person of your perceptions as they apply the technique and share details of the changes and the success that you are actually witnessing.

6. Give a homework assignment to repeat this process a certain number of times a day. This turns the power and the magic back to each person which is where it should be in the first place.

7. Ask them to listen to the recording multiple times.

Let's look at each component in more detail.

**1. Accurately describe the appearance and the sensations of the area of disease.** Every time I fail to mention some element of psychic insight to an individual, I regret it. The more informed a person is, the more information they have to work with to heal. Some of the information that you pick up will be, quite frankly, ugly. However, if you share the ugliness in a sensitive, kind, and loving manner, people will be more able to receive it. If you do not share it accurately, how will you then create an accurate healing assignment?

**2. See and especially feel each person in their healthiest and most vital state of being, however ill they are in the present moment.** Even as you witness "the good, the bad and the ugly," you must also maintain the vision and the sensation of wholeness and the wonderment of health-filled vitality. If you cannot hold that rich, healing energy for the person sitting before you, how can you guide them toward that goal? You are offering your energetic awareness during a medical intuition session. Your energy intermingles with each person you come in contact with. When you powerfully hold the visions and perceptions of robust health, you provide them with a foundation to learn, grow, and heal.

**3. Create a specific energetic experience that begins an energetic alteration toward healing.** The experience includes thinking, feeling, and visualizing in a certain manner. You are creating the energy experience through intuitive hits that pop into your mind. The energy experience comes from your spirit specialty guide.

Let me explain this in more detail. I create a specific energetic exercise at the close of the session based on a troubled spot that I just scanned. For example, I was doing a reading with a woman who had the most extraordinary, beautiful, shimmering aura I had ever witnessed. All I could see throughout her entire body was iridescent glimmering rainbows. I was immediately drawn like a magnet to her liver, which looked like rotten meat.

At the end of her session, I gave her an energy assignment. I asked her to think of a color that she loved and to fill her liver with that color and that energy. I pointed out to her where the liver is and asked her to inhale as usual but to also imagine her liver inhaling at the same time. I emphasized that she imagine the *feel* of her liver taking in breath and color and it moving through her abdomen into her liver.

### Vibrational Colors for Healing

The following is a guideline for deciding which color to use for certain physical issues. Chose a certain color for its healing qualities and teach your client how to visualize and also imagine feeling the colors within their body.

Sometimes Spirit gives me a certain color for the energy assignment, but I often receive directions to allow the person to choose a color. I do ask that it be clear and bright or even sparkling. I ask the person to feel the color that they picked and how it feels different from other colors. Colors are so much more than just colors. Each color is a distinct electrical frequency and carries a specific vibration.

I will also ask them to practice during the session so they experience the exercise before I close the session. I psychically watch the client, and I can tell if they are doing it correctly. It is amazing to see their energy field immediately change before my eyes. I of course tell them how they are indeed altering their own body and energy. Most people are delighted to know they can do this and have confirmation that it is happening already.

| Red | builds vitality, brings warmth to cold areas |
|---|---|
| Orange | good for all issues regarding elimination of toxins in kidneys, bladder, and lymph system |
| Yellow | builds warmth, increases sense of one's own individuality, good for issues regarding skin and bone conditions |

| Green | renewal, regeneration, decongestant, disinfectant |
|-------|-----------------------------------------------------|
| Blue | soothing in general, good for anxiety and inflammation, decreases fevers |
| Purple/Violet | breaks up energetic blocks, cleanses, builds a positive response for all mental and physical situations |

**4. Inform each person how to put the energy assignment into action.** Sensitively point out the negative descriptive words that they have used during the session and help them reframe those words into the positive. Ask the person to remember the feeling of love and to recreate the feeling of love right now. Ask them to *feel* the difference of positive words and emotions. I then direct the person to think and feel a certain color that they love.

Any color is fine as long as it is clear and bright. No matter where the illness is located I ask them to breathe that color into the area of the body that is affected. It is vital to ask them to imagine the *feel* of a color. For example, red, yellow, and orange might feel like a warm, cozy fire in a fireplace, while blues and greens will feel cool and crisp.

Inform them that it will always feel like they are simply dreaming it up. Ask them to imagine pulling in the bright, clear color into the place of illness and breaking up the density that has accumulated there.

**5. Practice all homework assignments during the session and watch their energetic field and body as they apply the technique.** Inform them how they are immediately changing their own energy field and what you are aware of as it happens. If their energy is not changing for the better and they are struggling, encourage them to continue and offer assistance to push the energy through. Let them know the tiniest changes you can see. Encourage each person to continue the energy assignment every day at home and to notice improvements.

Sometimes I give an assignment to take a tiny bit of action in life that is different than what they are doing. For instance, if the throat chakra is thick, dense, with little flow, I will ask the person to speak out more and let others simply know their likes or dislikes about certain restaurants or a certain topic. It is important that the assignment be very small, nonthreatening, and doable so the person is confident that they can do it and not fail. If the assignment is too large or too important, your client will fail to do it and thus reinforce their issue rather than heal it.

Ask them to repeat the energetic process that you and your specialty guide came up with. Giving a homework assignment gives each person a feeling of control and doing something positive for themselves. Tell people not to make this another task or another job to do because that only generates negative energy again.

**6. Give a homework assignment to repeat this process a certain number of times a day.** The energy homework needs to be incorporated throughout the day as each person continues on with their life. You might ask them, for example, to do their homework as they shower or as they watch TV. Ask them to do it at least three times per day. In this way, I reinforce an awareness of the individual's responsibility by giving each person specific homework to do each day.

Do not fall into the trap of checking with them later to see if they followed through with their homework or not. It is up to them, not you, to live their life. All we can do is give the information and the guidance when asked, but it is up to them to do it. Giving them homework turns the power and the magic back to each person, which is where it should be in the first place. The homework consists of reinforcing the information that you have given them to enhance their mindfulness about their own being. The homework also gives them an action to take if they choose to do it or not. The action is specifically based on a problem that you just perceived. It is often an energy assignment to feel and experience a higher vibrational color than how the energy is appearing at the time of the reading.

**7. Ask them to listen to the recording of the session many times** to assist them in staying on track for their health. In other words, you are asking them to reinforce and remember the detailed information that you shared about their health and their struggles. By frequently listening to the recording, you are asking them to stay alert regarding their own body, mind, and spirit and some of the issues that tend to bring trouble and resistance into their lives. If the person is in your office, you can download the recording onto a CD and hand it to them on the way out the door. If you are giving a phone reading you can send the recording via email by using a program such Sugarsync or Dropbox. Due to the technology age that we live in, more people will ask you to email the recording to them even if they are in your office.

The professional intuitive now has different ways to offer sessions to others. Many do the traditional face-to-face readings. Many readings are done over the phone and the intuitive never actually sees the person eye to eye. Now with the Internet opening up the world in infinite ways, some readings are done with a webcam. I am told that some readings are done through email and no one even hears the other's voice. Technology has opened up the world for the medical intuitive and like myself, you may find yourself giving readings all over the world. As we expand, the world expands and our interpersonal connections are uniting a global community.

When someone receives a medical intuitive reading from you, they will sometimes feel as if they stepped into magic. They will be amazed at your insights and the intimate details that you tell them. They will feel a sincere wonderment about it all. Do you realize that this amazed wonderment can also cause them to believe that you are the authority? If you maintain this level of authority with your clients, you will be giving them the ultimate information and the ultimate knowledge. They are the creator of their life and they are the creator of the quality of their life. Most people do not realize that they can have their own magic and can live it.

**Take Medical Intuition into Your World**

Where and how does one begin as a medical intuitive? You can begin with exploring this ability and awareness. By exploring I mean that you now need to discover how you perceive and what you perceive. In other words, how are you as an individual picking up this information? What senses are your strongest and what does the information look like, feel like, sound like, or smell like? How do you pick up your sense of knowing?

I am sitting in a public library as I write this section of the book. I am looking at twelve people that I do not know, but they are twelve people I could intuitively ask permission to scan. I remind you again and again to ask permission first. Practice not only on people around you but practice on people at a distance as well. Remember that you must ask for permission verbally or psychically.

If you receive the sensations of no in any way, shape, or form, you must honor that person's refusal no matter what. But when you receive a yes, begin taking the steps for medical intuition. Each person you come across is an opportunity to practice your medical intuition and also your psychic awareness of asking for permission to scan the human body.

Good counselors never counsel their own family members because they are too emotionally involved to give healthy guidance. It is the same for the medical intuitive's family. When practicing with a family member, I recommend that you direct your intent to only look at the illness itself and not delve deeper into their entire story. You cannot reach the clarity of the unbiased, neutral observer regarding the entire story of a relative. Look only at the illness to understand how it appears and what your senses tell you about it. You are in control of what you do and where you do it.

Practice with people that you know the least about. You will discover that you feel clearer about your psychic information. When you do not have anything personally invested, you have less emotion to get in the way. Remember that most emotions carry a thicker, heavier frequency that hinders and drags down the finer, more perceptive spirit mind. The more you practice on acquaintances or people you know little about, the purer your information will be.

As you do more and more medical intuitive readings you will come across another situation within a session. The person you are scanning might also, at some point, ask you to do a quick evaluation of someone they know. It might be this person's spouse or a neighbor. When this first happened to me I was not sure what to do, but then I heard the word "permission." So even though that person was not present, I asked for permission before continuing on.

For example, I was working with a dear woman on the East Coast over the phone. She was so stressed over her boyfriend who recently suffered an accident. She asked me to check in with him to evaluate his condition. I informed her that I needed to ask him for permission and if I got a refusal from him, I must honor it. She said she understood.

I asked for his first name only, then rhythmically repeated his name over in my mind and as I did that I looked around in her energy field for him. As soon as I felt this man give me permission, I felt a sinking feeling in my own body as if gravity was forcing me down inside of myself. I felt a sensation of being lost. Then a sharp pain shot through my head. It began at the top of my head and slightly to the right, bursting at an angle through my head to my right eye and upper lip.

As I described all these things, this dear woman began to cry uncontrollably, stating that his injuries damaged the right side of his brain and he had a large bruise around his right eye. She went on to say that he was not the same person he was six weeks ago. He often seemed blank or lost and acted and talked as if he were around ten years old.

When she asked me if he would recover, I sat and waited to see what popped into my awareness about her question. I could not perceive any changes happening in the future. Nothing moved in the images I saw. I told her that intuitives can only perceive the strongest energy current flowing out into the future and that we always have the option to alter, change, and make new choices for the future. "It is not set in stone," I reinforced. She then validated my impressions, stating that his physician had already documented the future for her boyfriend was exactly the same as I had stated.

Be careful when your client asks you to check in on another individual. I emphasize that I must intuitively receive permission from the other person before I divulge any information. I *never* share the possibility of an approaching death no matter what. I always want to give my client and the other person some hope, not shatter their hopes. *Always* strongly emphasize that intuitives can only receive what is strongest in one's energy field at the moment the intuitive does the scan. Tell your client the following: Nothing is ever set in stone in any way. There are forever an uncountable number of possibilities and choices in one's life every minute.

Read the information in this book over and over to assimilate and incorporate medical intuition into your being. Log your process and watch it develop. Remember that we are born and wired to do this very thing for each other. As each of us develops our personal awareness we assist the universe to develop as well.

The ancient healers, medicine men, herbalists, and seers have been assessing the human condition since the beginning of time. We are not creating anything new as we acknowledge the innate abilities of our present bodymind. These abilities are more than gifts. They are natural talents that we have been given from our source. We are merely remembering and living the empowerment that is innate within the human experience.

Our Universe is changing, expanding, and transforming. We are literally stepping into a new age of enlightenment. We utilize the collective intelligence of the Internet, but we can also utilize the collective intelligence of Source. Our medical system is astounding at finding and diagnosing disease, but discovering how the disease developed or what factors created it seems nonexistent.

Western medicine discovers illness and treats it but does not discover the cause. Medical intuition assesses the symptoms but ventures beyond the symptoms and uncovers the cause. Medical intuition understands that if the bodymind can help create illness, it can also create wellness.

Traditional healthcare and the medical intuitive can work together in true harmony. The healthcare system simply needs to understand our value as medically based intuitives. We can function as valued co-creators of wellness, not competitors against the medical field. Can you even imagine the domino effect for our world when medical intuitives are in every town, every city and state, and every country? Collectively, we can make quantum leaps in knowledge for the betterment of human health.

I am driven to teach medical intuition around the world. My goal is to pass this on to everyone who is ready to receive it. When there are medical intuitives in every city, in every country, the allopathic medical world will notice. When the medical intuitive openly works in conjunction with physicians and not against them, they will notice. Medical intuition is the missing piece of the enormous healthcare puzzle. There is a place for us in the existing healthcare world.

The medical intuitive accesses the intimate, personal story that each of us carries within our body and our energy field. Each story is dramatically unique, containing a myriad of facets, people, experiences, and development. Hold this skill in an honored place in your heart and it will not forsake you.

The medical intuitive lives a life of knowing and perceiving with x-ray eyes of the soul.

Blessings to you forever,

Tina Zion

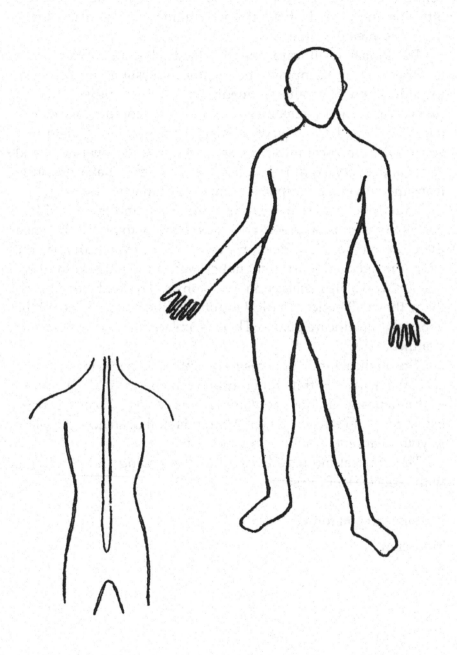

# Suggested Reading

*The Amazing Power of Deliberate Intent: Living the Art of Allowing* by Esther Hicks and Jerry Hicks

*Ask Your Guides: Connecting to Your Divine Support System* by Sonia Choquette

*The Book of Awakening* by Mark Nepo

*Destiny of Souls* by Michael Newton, PhD

*The Encyclopedic Psychic Dictionary* by June Bletzer, PhD

*The Energy Healing Experiments: Science Reveals Our Natural Power to Heal* by Gary Schwartz, PhD

*Everything You Need to Know to Feel Go(o)d* by Candace Pert, PhD

*Fabric of the Cosmos: Space, Time and the Texture of Reality* by Brian Greene

*Hands of Light* by Barbara Brennan

*Heal Your Body* by Louise Hay

*Journey of Souls* by Michael Newton, PhD

*The Living Energy Universe: A Fundamental Discovery that Transforms Science and Medicine* by Gary Schwartz, PhD

*Memories of the Afterlife: Life Between Lives Stories of Personal Transformation* by Michael Newton, PhD (Tina is a contributing author in this book)

*Molecules of Emotion* by Candace Pert, PhD

*The Sacred Promise: How Science is Discovering Spirit's Collaboration with Us in Our Daily Lives* by Gary Schwartz, PhD

*Second Sight* by Judith Orloft

*Vibrational Medicine* by Richard Gerber, MD

*The Vortex: Where the Law of Attraction Assembles All Cooperative Relationships* by Esther Hicks and Jerry Hicks

*When Ghosts Speak* by Mary Ann Winkowsky

# About the Author

**To continue your medical intuition training check out Tina's new book.** *Advanced Medical Intuition: 6 Underlying Causes of Illness and Unique Healing Methods.*

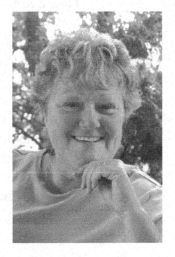

**TINA M. ZION** is a fourth generation intuitive medium, specializing in medical intuition and teaching it internationally. She has worked in the mental health field as a registered nurse with a national board specialty certification in mental health nursing from the American Nurses Credentialing Association. Tina is a Gestalt trained counselor, graduating from the Indianapolis Gestalt Institute in 1997. She received her certification in clinical hypnotherapy from the American Council of Hypnotist Examiners in 1985, and was specialized in past life regressions and certified through the Michael Newton Institute for Life Between Life Regressions. She is the now an internationally known best-selling author of *Advanced Medical Intuition, The Reiki Teacher's Manual* and is a contributing author in Newton's book, *Memories of the Afterlife.*

Tina no longer offers individual readings. Her private practice now specifically focuses on teaching her workshop "Become a Medical Intuitive: Seeing with X-Ray Eyes" and working with individuals to enhance their natural intuitive skills.

**Tina Zion offers the following to you:**

- **Medical Intuition: Seeing with X-Ray Eyes**
  Tina presents her workshop all over the world. Contact Tina to host her workshop in your area or in your country.

- **Intuition Mentoring** through Skype, the phone, or in person. The focus of each session is to build and empower your personal abilities and skills. Tina does not have a set agenda for your sessions. Each session focuses on your wishes, needs, or issues regarding your intuitive development.

Tina's website is www.livingawareinc.com

## Book Cover by Corey Ford

Corey Ford has worked in oil, pastel, acrylic, pencil and digital art. Her fine art paintings are in private collections throughout the United States and her digital paintings are used on a worldwide basis in advertising, book, CD, and DVD covers, company logos, and wall murals. She is always striving to put her visions into art and finding the best way to achieve this. Her art is always evolving and changing as the years go by but her love for it is eternal.

Corey's website is www.coreyfordgallery.com

## Diagrams by Jacqueline Rogers

Jacqueline Rogers is an illustrator of many books, mostly for children. You can see more of her work on her website, www.jacquelinerogers.com